Health, Illness, and
Medical Care in Japan

CONTRIBUTORS

CHRISTIE W. KIEFER
University of California, San Francisco

MARGARET LOCK
McGill University

SUSAN ORPETT LONG
John Carroll University

EDWARD NORBECK
Rice University

DAVID K. REYNOLDS
ToDo Institute and Health Center Pacific

NANCY R. ROSENBERGER
Emory University

WILLIAM E. STESLICKE
University of South Florida

This book is based on a conference sponsored by the Joint Committee on Japanese Studies of the American Council of Learned Societies and the Social Science Research Council.

Health, Illness, and Medical Care in Japan

Cultural and Social Dimensions

*Edited by Edward Norbeck
and Margaret Lock*

 University of Hawaii Press • HONOLULU

© 1987 University of Hawaii Press
All rights reserved
Manufactured in the United States of America

Library of Congress Cataloging-in-Publication Data

Health, illness, and medical care in Japan.

   Revised and edited papers given at the American
Anthropological Association Meeting held in Chicago in
Nov., 1983; sponsored by the Joint Committee on Japanese
Studies of the American Council of Learned Societies and
the Social Science Research Council.
   Includes bibliographies and index.
   1. Social medicine—Japan—Congresses.   2.   Public
health—Japan—Congresses.   I.   Norbeck, Edward,
1915–   .   II.   Lock, Margaret M.   III.   American
Anthropological Association. Meeting (82nd : 1983 :
Chicago, Ill.)   IV.   Joint Committee on Japanese Studies.
[DNLM: 1.   Delivery of Health Care—Japan—congresses.
2.   Health Policy—Japan—congresses. W 84 JJ3 H4]
RA418.3.J3H43   1987   362.1'0952   87–10753
ISBN 0–8428–1102–X

To the memory of Bill Lebra

CONTENTS

FOREWORD

In my file of miscellaneous materials there is a color reproduction of a painting that epitomizes the common view of the relationship between modern biomedicine and the indigenous medical systems it has encountered. Identified only as taken from a 1930s Soviet publication, *Paintings by Yakut Artists,* it shows an interior scene. On a platform bed, covered by an animal skin throw, lies a woman with oriental features and long black hair. In a dark corner near the foot of the bed stand a small boy and an old man whose features register anxiety and resignation, respectively. At the back of the room, looking out sternly from under a fur-lined parka, is a man who seems to be the patient's husband. For patient she is. Standing full center is the sturdy figure of a woman in the process of removing a heavy fur outercoat to reveal her gleaming white nurse's uniform. She stands, obviously having been brought to the house by the husband, purposefully and powerfully delineated, looking toward the patient. Her features are Caucasian, her short hair, light brown. She is placed between the bed and a dark figure of a man whose posture suggests that he has been pushed aside. His features, like those of all the family members, are oriental, his long hair, jet black. Clad in full regalia and holding a skin drum and stick, he has been thrust into semidarkness. The painting, by one A. N. Ossipov, is entitled *The Expulsion of the Shaman.* It might well have been subtitled "Superstition Eclipsed by the Light of Reason."

Readers of the contributions to this volume will soon discover that the allegory so carefully worked out by the Soviet artist could hardly be less appropriate to the contemporary Japanese medical scene. In one way or another every essay reveals how consistently and thoroughly interwoven are the several systems by means of which the Japanese define health and the ways in which illness can be treated. Modern biomedical scientific practice was in fact built on the existing structure of the practice of what is loosely called "Chinese medicine." The Meiji government, in the late nineteenth century, did indeed sponsor the establishment of Western biomedical science, as the Soviet government was to do in its turn, but in Japan no move was made to stamp out the indigenous system already in place. The authorities controlled its practice, to be sure, but a pluralistic system has flourished for over a century. Over the years a degree of integration has taken place so that the recent boom in the use of herbal medicines is traceable in part to its promotion by Japan's great pharmaceutical houses. Thus, the Japanese—ever concerned with health and given to equating illness with disorder—enjoy the benefits of medical pluralism and increasingly exploit its diversity.

There is yet another major emphasis in these essays that greatly aids our understanding of how such systems work. In Japan, as in most—perhaps all—other societies today, the professionally given definitions of health, illness, and therapy are all in important ways shaped by social and cultural beliefs concerning the body, the concept of the self and identity, and the relationship of the individual to society. Folk or popular medical knowledge and assumptions are deeply implicated in the professional biomedical definitions of proper health maintenance, symptoms of illness, and effective treatment of them. We would expect to find such cultural influences in, say, the psychotherapies, but the authors show similar interweaving of social and cultural factors in what are usually seen as purely technical medical decisions such as length of hospital stay, degree of intrusiveness of treatment, and analysis of the origins of the multiplying syndromes so widely reported in the Japanese press. That such decisions are strongly influenced by the notion that the primary responsibility for health and the successful treatment of illness rests squarely on the individual and members of the immediate social group —particularly the family—is only one of the many findings reported here that reveals how society and culture figure in the operation of seemingly autonomous technical domains.

What is true for Japan is equally true for other societies where indigenous medical systems are fused with biomedicine. If these papers successfully defend that proposition, as I believe they do, then we are in the authors' debt for giving us one more example of the essential failure of the convergence model of modernization. That model holds that we are all tending in the same direction and says, in effect, that the expulsion of the shaman by the nurse is the inevitable outcome of the clash of medical systems in all societies. If the argument were valid, the Japanese medical scene by rights ought to be far less variegated and complex than it is after more than a century of full-scale adoption of alien biomedical teaching and practice. What has happened instead is the establishment of a pluralistic medical system strongly grounded in Japanese conceptions of the nature of men and women, the sources of their physical and psychological well-being, and the treatable causes of ill-health and disorder. Insofar as these considerations are socially and culturally specific, the resulting medical system is identifiably Japanese. To the degree that all medical systems are incorporative rather than exclusive, the contributions to this volume clearly signal the necessity to look more closely at our own.

Robert J. Smith
Cornell University

ACKNOWLEDGMENTS

An expression of hearty thanks is due to the Social Science Research Council, the moving spirit in the preparation of this volume. The council provided the original inspiration and the funds for a planning meeting on themes relating to Japanese health and illness that was organized by Edward Norbeck and held at Rice University. Several pertinent topics were selected as especially suitable for further elaboration and presentation as papers at the American Anthropological Association Meeting held in Chicago in November 1983. The contents of this volume, revised versions of the papers given at that meeting, have benefited from the critical discussion given by George De Vos and Michael Reich at the panel presentation and by editing from Edward Norbeck. The authors would also like to thank the several anonymous referees for their helpful comments and the University of Hawaii Press for a magnificent job of editing and production.

Introduction: Health and Medical Care as Cultural and Social Phenomena

MARGARET LOCK

If human beings could be improved like oxen,
I suppose it would be possible after some years for
the Japanese to boast physiques as powerful as
the Westerners', to be strong, free from illness,
and economical human beings, any one of whom
can do the work of three men of today. But I
wonder if in that case the qualities of the special
inborn character of the Japanese people would
still exist. I doubt it somehow.
   —Masaoka Shiki, *Bokujū itteki* (A drop
    of ink), 1901

The comparative study of health and illness has proved to be, in recent years, a rich source for the cross-fertilization of ideas among the social sciences. This, in turn, has led to some new conceptualizations about how best to go about conducting research and interpreting data.

Several factors have contributed to the emergence of an interdisciplinary approach to the analysis of health care. Over the past thirty years, and with increasing vigor of late, the subdiscipline known as the sociology of knowledge, drawing primarily on philosophical theory and often using the small-sample ethnographic methods of anthropology, has developed a rigorous critique of the notion that the scientific method is a value-free endeavor. The way has been opened for the analysis of biomedicine as a cultural product, and the sociologist Freidson was one of the first to undertake such a study. Since the publication of Freidson's *Profession of Medicine* in 1970, numerous critical studies representing a range of perspectives have appeared. Navarro's presentation (1976) of the Marxist view of the links between capitalism and biomedicine and Illich's well-known book (1976) focusing on the shortcomings of the medical profession itself are two examples; a third is McKeown's sober and carefully researched study (1976) attributing improved health in late

1

nineteenth and early twentieth-century Europe mainly to improved nutritional status and public health measures and not to services provided by the medical profession. It is not altogether surprising that, concurrent with these developments, a flood of popular interest in alternative and exotic health care systems emerged, an interest partially fueled by the research of anthropologists into comparative medical systems and in which Asian medicine figured prominently (see, for example, Kleinman 1979; Leslie 1976; Lock 1980).

Many researchers who wish to account adequately for the generation of medical knowledge and the institutionalization and practice of medicine, whether in a nonliterate or a complex society, have gradually come to see that most of the traditional, discipline-confined approaches used in the social sciences are too narrow. The work of both the physician and the shaman is invariably modified by political forces. The "popular" cultural construction of ideas about the cosmos and the relationship of people to nature and the spirit world as well as ideas about birth, death, gender, human anatomy, physiology, nutrition, body boundaries, social identity, the nature of emotions, normality and abnormality, early socialization, and so on, all contribute to shared ideas in any one medical tradition. Members participating in any tradition, whether they are ordinary people or professionals, help to sustain and change these ideas.

"Professional" beliefs about health, preventive medicine, and etiology of illnesses and their nosology and therapy, all of which form the corpus of esoteric medical knowledge, including biomedicine, are everywhere partially structured by popular medical knowledge (Helman 1978; Hahn and Gaines 1985) and are the product of a particular historical, institutional, and political setting. This situation is made more complex because in most parts of the world today societies have been exposed to at least one and often two major, literate medical traditions, the ideas of which have been superimposed, often over the course of hundreds of years, upon an indigenous nonliterate medical tradition. A state of pluralism is normal but is rarely explicitly recognized as such by members of a society. It is only the fastidious historian or anthropologist who takes the trouble to tease out the origins of various medical ideas.

Thus, medically related conceptions are embedded in a mesh of cultural concepts, what Peter Worsley (1982) has called a "metamedical" framework. Isolation and study of components such as a "medical system" or "tradition," a hospital, a clinic, or a healing session, are artificially bounded units superimposed by the social scientist who undertakes the analysis. It is, of course, necessary to create some sort of controllable units in order to collect and analyze data. It is also essential, however, that preconceived notions about the complete separation of, for example, biomedical knowledge and religious or political beliefs or biomedical practice and ritual or magic be carefully scrutinized and not assumed a priori as natural and inevitable.

The Study of Health and Illness in Japan

We have come a considerable distance from the first publication by a Westerner of what could be loosely classified as a study into health care in Japan. In the thirties a large part of a Ciba symposium on bathing was devoted to the therapeutic nature of Japanese baths (Martin 1939). Since that time various ethnographies have recorded a great deal of information that contributes both to our understanding of contemporary behavior in connection with health and illness and to our knowledge about the metamedical framework in Japan (see Beardsley, Hall, and Ward 1959; Embree 1939; Norbeck 1954; Smith 1978). Research focusing on religious beliefs, such as that by Smith (1974), Lebra (1976b), and Yoshida (1967), has been particularly important in this respect. Contributions by psychological anthropologists and psychiatrists (Caudill 1976; DeVos 1973; Doi 1973; Doi 1986) have also been invaluable in laying the groundwork for a culturally informed analysis of Japanese medical ideas. The work of scholars such as Nakane (1970) and Fukutake (1980) on social organization in Japan provides important points of departure for an analysis of the institutionalized health care system.

The collection of writings in this volume represents only a portion of the recent social science research on health, illness, and healing in Japan. The vast literature on epidemiology and on quantitative approaches to the analysis of the Japanese health care complex (see, for example, Ikegami 1980; Munakata 1986; Yamamoto 1978; Yamamoto and Ohmura 1975), though not represented in this collection, is referred to in many of the essays in this volume, especially that by William Steslicke. There is also a literature produced mainly by medical professionals but also by some social scientists that has a direct bearing on applied medical care and that focuses largely on the encounter between health care professionals and patients (see, for example, Ikemi et al. 1980). This topic is not dealt with here because, rather than remaining within the narrow scientific perspective almost invariably adopted in modern medical and epidemiological circles, the contributors to this volume have undertaken studies *of* rather than *in* medicine and its related realms. In other words, despite the fact that one of us, David Reynolds, is both a trained social scientist and a medical practitioner, we have retained in the studies that follow a perspective that is separate and analytical rather than one that is primarily applied. Even within this perspective, however, the topics are necessarily limited, and extremely important areas are left unexamined in this particular volume, including contemporary religious beliefs and practices and their relationship to healing (Davis 1980; Lebra 1982; Yoshida 1984); connections between indigenous categories of thought and current health beliefs and practices (Lock 1982b; Ohnuki-Tierney 1984); ideas about contraception and reproduction (Coleman 1983); suicide (Iga et al. 1978; Iga 1986); industrial pollution and related problems (McKean 1981; Reich 1984); the "culture," social organization, and education of health care personnel (Long 1980, 1984, 1986); the traditional literate medical tradition (Lock 1980); and historical studies on health-related issues (Smith 1977).

What is unusual about this collection of essays is that a broad range of topics relating to health and illness are addressed in a number of ways by one political scientist and five anthropologists, none of whom are limited by the theories of their own disciplines but who draw upon all of the social sciences to a greater or lesser degree in an attempt to portray some fragments of the extraordinarily complex picture that is modern Japan.

The topic chosen teaches us about an aspect of Japanese culture that has not been well documented until recently. In so doing, many of the critical dilemmas and paradoxes that plague the society as it proceeds apace with industrial expansion and economic growth are exposed through a new lens. These studies in health and illness reveal from a unique vantage point the way in which the process of modernization has become encoded into and expressed through the body, at times to its benefit but at other times to its detriment.

The Health Care Complex

William Steslicke, in his overview of the Japanese health care system, contrasts what he terms the "health miracle" (the remarkable improvements in life expectancy and infant mortality) with costs to health (diseases caused by environmental pollution and the increased incidence of heart disease and cancer, among many other problems). Steslicke points out that the Japanese, like people of other industrial nations, have become "health care consumers," who expect and demand the ready availability of high-technology professionalized medical services. While local family practitioners, acupuncturists, and practitioners of massage remain fully occupied, nevertheless, a great demand is placed on large centrally located hospitals. It is not unusual to see people queuing up at the entrances of hospital outpatient departments beginning at six o'clock in the morning in order to be among the first patients to be seen when the doors open at nine. Most women, for example, now prefer to give birth in hospitals where use is made of technology such as fetal monitors, leading to a decline in the use of obstetrician/gynecologists who run their own small, private clinics. This trend, combined with an increased use of contraception and hence a reduction in the abortion rate, has caused some of these private practitioners to go out of business (Lock 1987).

Susan Long and William Steslicke both stress the power of the Japanese government in shaping the implementation of medical care, a situation that makes Japan more comparable with European countries or Canada than with the United States. Steslicke, who has done more than anyone over the years to describe and analyze for the English-speaking audience the intricacies of the Japanese medical care complex, summarizes the system thus: the bulk of medical care is provided by the "private sector," where the delivery of services is highly competitive leading to redundancy in some areas. The average length of stay in hospitals is 38.3 days as opposed to 8 days in the United States. Steslicke suggests that this can be explained in part by the fact that hospitals are not separated into acute and chronic care facilities, as they are in North America. Other factors implicated by Steslicke are the structure of health insurance plans in Japan, which allows for more generous hospital stays, and cultural ideas about the importance of nurturance and rest during illness (see also Lebra 1976a; Lock 1980; Kiefer, this volume).

One feature of the Japanese medical system that creates chronic policy problems is the combining of a predominately private, fee-for-service, physician-centered system of care with a compulsory health insurance system (Abe 1985; Steslicke 1982a). Although the health insurance system is universal, many people do not use it and are covered instead by private policies not only for illness but for health-related benefits such as retirement funding. These private policies, which are offered to employees of large businesses, provide much better coverage than do the government-managed plans to which owners and employees of small businesses and poorer members of society such as the elderly and unemployed tend to belong. This two-tiered system is often the target of policy reform but so far with little success (Steslicke 1982c).

The "closed-staff" system in Japanese hospitals that are organized as self-contained units limits the possibility for referrals and for liaison work. This system also encourages each hospital to be comprehensive and in competition with other hospitals for acquisition of the latest technology, with the result that the quality of care may vary widely (Niki 1985). This same system contributes to poor coordination and continuity of services from primary to specialized care, little concern with rehabilitation and prevention, and inadequate regional health care planning. In an attempt to rectify some of the shortcomings of the closed-staff system, certain well-publicized experimental projects have been undertaken. Two of these are described by Christie Kiefer in this volume. Other projects designed in part to provide possible models for large-scale changes in the future include the 35-year-old primary health care experiment run out of Saku hospital in Nagano prefecture (Abrams 1979; Nishirai 1983), a community health experiment being conducted seventy kilometers north of Tokyo (Miyasaka 1971), and the much more recent privately funded Life Planning Center, founded by a Tokyo physician and created to increase public awareness of preventive health care.

Steslicke also points out that although most Japanese physicians are trained as specialists, by far the majority of them work as general practitioners operating their own small private practice. It is widely recognized that a fee-for-service system encourages aggressive medical practice. A carefully controlled study published in 1976 demonstrated how an annual increase in the rate of appendectomy in Japan (up to three times that of England) was directly correlated to the institution of the fee-for-service system (Yoshida and Yoshida 1976).

One of the most controversial features of the system is that physicians are permitted to both dispense and prescribe drugs, a situation that is clearly linked with excessive use of medication in Japan (Abe 1985). Herbal medication has recently been introduced into the picture; one or two drug companies have begun to promote attractively packaged traditional herbal medication among physicians, who are now legally able to receive reimbursement for its prescription. It is reported that over two-thirds of all Japanese physicians prescribe herbal medication at times, some with great frequency (*Nikkei Medical* 1981). This means that traditional medicine has entered the world of big business, a change that has enormous implications for both modern and traditional medicinal practice (Lock 1984b; and see Long, this volume).

Steslicke's chapter describes the ongoing efforts at cost containment in the health care system today, the roles of the various government agencies in this process, and the complex relationship of these agencies to the medical profession and to the "health care industry" composed primarily of drug companies and manufacturers of medical technology. He points out that policymakers in future will have to face up to a much more demanding Japanese public, a public that has a growing sense of entitlement to good care. He also predicts that the health of the public will increasingly be pitted against the interests of those officials in government who are concerned more with fiscal than physical health, and that the Japan Medical Association, at present undergoing a period of reorganization, could be a wild card in the delicate process of reform.

The Process of Medicalization

The topic of medicalization comes up in all but one of the contributions to this volume. Early studies on the process of medicalization (mostly in the United States and Britain) tended to emphasize the role of the medical profession, which some critics believe actively creates a market for its services principally by redefining certain behaviors and problems as diseases (Freidson 1970; Zola 1978).

There have been four critical lines of thought in the past few years that have broadened our understanding of the process of medicalization. The first proposes that the practice of medicine is a reflection of the organization and values of society at large and that members of the medical profession are themselves members of particular cultures, societies, and political systems. Related to this is the second point, graphically illustrated in Susan Long's chapter in this volume, that professional interests and power are seriously curtailed by government intervention, the interests of which are often at odds with those of the profession.

Third, the medical profession is not a uniform, hegemonic institution; rather, it is made up of a variety of interest groups that form, to some extent, independent bases of power. In Japan there are constant tensions between national and regional medical organizations. Tensions also exist among speciality groups and between clinicians and researchers, salaried hospital-based and private practitioners, rural and urban practitioners, and M.D.s practicing traditional medicine and those practicing biomedicine. In characteristic Japanese fashion, factions form behind each of these interest groups and become enmeshed in a web of conflicting and competing interests. This leads to a very complex situation, which has not yet received sufficient analytic attention, although Susan Long's work has consistently made some important contributions in this respect.

The final point to be noted in connection with the process of medicalization is that there has to be a cooperative public willing to visit physicians, sit in waiting rooms, and stay in hospital beds. Probably every Westerner who has observed the implementation of medical care in Japan has been struck by how readily the Japanese public makes use of health care facilities, physicians, and medication (a topic that, though statistically documented [Okino 1978], awaits fuller analysis). What also strikes an outsider is the extreme time pressure that physicians work under (on average, three minutes per patient), due largely to the structure of payment for their work. The payment structure also encourages physicians to focus on physical interventions, since they are reimbursed only for the procedures they perform. These factors, along with various cultural reasons of long historical tradition (Lock 1980; Ohnuki-Tierney 1984; Kiefer, this volume), produce a strong tendency for interactions between physicians and patients to be focused upon the physical body and the furnishing of treatment for it. Environmental, social, and psychological origins of illness tend to go unexamined in the offices of both physicians and traditional medical practitioners. This brings us fully into the purvue of medical anthropology and the cultural analysis of health and illness, which I will examine next in order to bring us back to the question of medicalization.

The Cultural Construction of Health and Illness

A recent flood of work in medical anthropology and sociology, some of which is inspired by Foucault (1973, 1979), has begun to question persistently the naive assumption that the body physical, because of its constitution from cells, molecules, and liquids, should be exempt from cultural analysis (Armstrong 1983; Bourdieu 1977; Comaroff 1985; Douglas 1970; Turner 1984). Contemporary research sets out to demonstrate that the body is socially and culturally produced and historically situated: it is both a part of nature and society but, at the same time, a representation of the way that nature and society are conceived. In order to understand how this is achieved in any given society, it is necessary to examine historical and contemporary cosmologies, ideas about the concept of self and the relationship of self and society, the "location" of the emotions in the physical body, the language of emotions, forms of expression of pain and discomfort and the meanings that are attributed to them, and ideas about body boundaries. An understanding of the nature of social relationships is also obviously crucial, as is an awareness of the culturally accepted means of expressing dissent and the use of the body as a symbolic medium for this purpose.

We are fortunate that so much literature is already available on many of these topics in Japan due to the rich tradition of Buddhist studies as well as psychological, psychoanalytic, and cultural anthropology. If concepts such as nurturance, loss, dependency, responsibility, and so on, are incorporated into the analysis, as is the case in the chapters by Reynolds and Kiefer in this volume, then continuities between the physical body, its cultural construction, and the larger social context become apparent.

The work of Caudill and Doi (1963) from more than twenty years ago produced significant results using this kind of approach. They demonstrated, among other things, how, because of cultural ideas about nonexposure of "real self" *(honne),* it is extremely difficult for Japanese patients to discuss their feelings with medical professionals. DeVos and Wagatsuma (1959) used the Thematic Apperception Test to show an association between introjected guilt and a concern about illness and death. They contrasted this situation with Hallowell's research with the Saulteaux, where sorcery is linked to the incidence of illness. (More recent studies over the past twenty years have shown a decline in the frequency of guilt feelings and suicidal ideation in association with illness in Japan [Shinfuku et al. 1973].) Lebra's studies (1974, 1976a, 1982) into religious groups and healing in Japan have consistently demonstrated that, in addition to paying attention to cognitive constructs, it is important to understand the symbolic presentation of self through the use of nonverbal communication in order to better understand the transactions that take place in healing ceremonies and between patients and their families. Reynolds (1976, 1980, 1981) in his portrayals of Japanese indigenous psychotherapeutic systems has given us a rich picture of a society that cultivates self-responsibility for the incidence of illnesses and that is disposed toward the use of techniques of introspection in psychotherapeutic healing. In a recent article Susan and Bruce Long (1982) use a symbolic interactionist approach to examine why Japanese physicians deem it unethical to reveal a "death sentence" of cancer. They discuss the way in which patients and family members immerse themselves in "proper" role behavior in order to collude with the physician in hiding the diagnosis.

One of the important contributions that Ohnuki-Tierney's research (1984) into Japanese medicine makes is to demonstrate that, by taking as the boundaries for our analyses the demarcations between medical systems as they are perceived by the Japanese themselves (which also happen to be the categories which make "common sense" to Western social scientists), we have often failed to show some very important features common to all types of Japanese health care. At the level of institutionalization there are indeed clear demarcations between folk, traditional literate, and biomedical systems of medicine (Lock 1982a; Long, this volume), but using a cultural and structural (in the Levi-Straussian sense of the term) analysis, it is possible to demonstrate, as does Ohnuki-Tierney, that there are certain concepts and values, such as those based upon ideas of purity and impurity, for example, that surface in a wide range of religious and medical settings, including modern hospitals. Doi's analysis (1986) of concepts such as *ura* "inside" and *omote* "outside" is also applicable in any setting. Although there is institutionalization and tolerance of pluralism (albeit with demarcations that weight distribution of power clearly in favor of the biomedical system today), at the level of the metamedical context made manifest in medical knowledge and practice, there is surprising consistency across many institutionalized boundaries.

In his chapter Reynolds points out some common features of all contemporary Japanese psychotherapeutic systems. The first is "specification," in which patients at intake interviews are required to give precise descriptions of self and symptoms. In his earlier work Reynolds discussed how many Japanese psychiatric patients tend to suffer from being overly focused upon themselves (this tendency is usually linked to Doi's [1973] famous discussion of the concept of *amae*). Because of this exaggerated self-focus, a second psychotherapeutic feature, "dissolving" self-focus, is central to most therapies in Japan. This is often accomplished by the use of techniques of introspection, just one example of "doing something" that is part of virtually all psychotherapies in Japan. Reynolds stresses that a large amount of time is spent in reflecting upon and restructuring relationships to authority figures, including that with the therapist if necessary (see also Tatara 1982). In conclusion he states that therapy always commences with an acceptance of the client as a worthy person.

Reynolds' discussion is particularly important because in it he also points out the differences in the therapies that he discusses. In a complex society such as Japan's, argues Reynolds, patients bring a variety of values and expectations to therapy, and he shows how there is flexibility and choice available to both therapists and patients.

In examining the plight of the elderly in modern Japan, Christie Kiefer examines political, economic, social, and cultural aspects of the problem. Using the key concept of responsibility toward family members, Kiefer analyzes the role played by women in looking after their elderly kin. He draws on the work of Caudill (1962), Doi (1973), and Lebra (1976a), who have all emphasized the passive helplessness *(amae)* manifested so often in social relationships in Japan and the caretaking response that it elicits *(amayakasu)*. The concepts of *amae* and *amayakasu* surface yet again in the behavior of the elderly and in their care. Kiefer demonstrates how these values contribute negatively (to a Western mind) to the condition of the elderly, encouraging the elderly to remain bedridden and offering no incentive for provision of rehabilitative services for them. Kiefer does not limit his analysis to cultural factors, however. He also points out the economic and political reasons for the continued encouragement of care for the elderly in their own homes as well as the negative historical associations on the part of both families and physicians in connection with nursing homes and the power of the medical profession in blocking the development of good nursing and paraprofessional services. Kiefer is careful to show that, though each of these factors can and should be analyzed in terms of the interests of powerful groups, they must also be viewed as partially the product of cultural values that the elite share with the vast majority of ordinary people. (For other recent studies on the elderly in Japan see articles by Steslicke, J. Campbell, Lock, Goldsmith, and R. Campbell, all in *Pacific Affairs* 1984.)

The first Western study on medical ethics in Japan was published in 1985. It should come as no surprise in light of the above discussion and the following essays, that the author of this study found consensus and deference to authority characteristic of the Japanese approach to ethical issues in health care (Feldman 1985). In this most recent field of medical activity there is a tendency among Western scholars to assume that ethically informed medical decisions are value free. However, this illustration from Japan demonstrates how, as with every other aspect of medical care, cultural patterning is inevitable.

Changing Symptom Patterns and the Epidemiology of Illness

The present volume does not suggest any reasons for, nor does it more than superficially discuss, the changing incidence of physical disease in Japan (see Steslicke, this volume, table 6). This is a topic worthy of serious interdisciplinary analysis, particularly in light of the findings by Marmot and Syme (1976) in their fifteen-year study of the incidence of coronary heart disease in Japanese Americans. After controlling for all the usual "hard" variables associated with the incidence of CHD, Marmot and Syme reach the conclusion that a large proportion of the variance must be explained by retention of traditional values during the process of acculturation after migration. The hasty abandonment of traditional values is associated, they find, with an increased risk of CHD (see also Cohen et al. 1979). These findings have been born out by studies in other cultural settings (see Scotch 1963, for example), and it would be interesting to undertake similar studies inside Japan itself.

Reynolds, in his contribution to this volume, discusses the way in which psychiatric symptoms have changed over the past forty years, including a decrease in neurotic complaints associated with a fear of blushing, *taijinkyofushō* (often regarded as a culture-bound syndrome [Tanaka-Matsumi 1979]). He cites an increase in neurotic depression and phobias in connection with eye contact and suggests some cultural reasons for these changes.

One of the major problems that arises in the assessment of psychiatric symptoms is the question of standardization in diagnostic techniques. Japan continues to provide a stern challenge to attempts to create a diagnostic system that is universally valid, and the problems of applying the American Psychiatric Association's latest classificatory system, DSM-III, are amply demonstrated by Honda (1983). It is not surprising that there is difficulty in standardizing psychiatric diagnosis, given the fact that the "mechanism" of the production of emotion is thought to be different in Japan than elsewhere (Tsunoda 1979); that language partially structures the means of expressing emotion (Beeman 1985); that the emotional "center" of the body in Japan was traditionally, at least, the abdomen *(hara)* and not the heart (Lock 1980); that, for example, Japanese tend to associate feelings of depression *(yūutsu)* with rain, clouds, and the dark, whereas Americans usually associate such feelings with despair and loneliness (Tanaka-Matsumi and Marsella 1976); and that there is repeated evidence, comparatively speaking, of a tendency to somatize (express through physical symptoms) rather than to verbalize about emotional states (Lock 1980, and this volume; Marsella 1980; Ohara 1973; Ohnuki-Tierney 1984; Shinfuku et al. 1973; Yoshimita, Kawano, and Takayama 1971).

Added to the complications that arise because of the cultural construction of emotion is the question of differential use and availability of mental health facilities. Mental illness is highly stigmatizing in Japan even today, whereas to consult with an ordinary physician about nonspecific functional complaints and to receive medication is completely acceptable. Relatively speaking, much greater use is made in Japan of medication and hospitalization for psychiatric problems than of psychotherapeutic methods (Ikegami 1980). These factors lead Western psychiatrists to believe that there is probably an underdiagnosis of problems such as depression, largely because general practitioners and internists (not only in Japan but throughout the world) do not easily recognize and diagnose depressive illnesses (Katon, Ries, and Kleinman 1984).

One other very important factor to note in the management of psychiatric illness is that diagnosis is a social process, the result of a negotiation between the presentation of symptoms by a patient and their assessment by a physician. Since physicians are as much a product of their cultures as are patients, it should not be surprising to find that there is considerable cross-cultural variation in psychiatric diagnosis. Marsella and his colleagues who work on the ongoing World Health Organization's multicenter study of depressive disorder (which includes Japan) conclude that, while the so-called core symptoms of depressive disorder can be found in many cultures, the full range of manifestations of depressive syndrome as it is conceived in the West is not universal. They stress that one cannot ignore the complex ways in which the incidence, experience of, and therapy for depression are culturally constructed. They caution that it is necessary first of all to distinguish clearly between prevalence and incidence studies, between normal and clinical populations, and between conceptualizations about feeling depressed and the actual manifestation and diagnosis of depressive syndrome (Marsella et al. 1985). The enormous difficulties in measurement of this disorder should not be underestimated, and further culturally informed research in Japan should produce invaluable data.

Social and Political Uses of Illness States

In the opening of her chapter on the social uses of menopause, Nancy Rosenberger emphasizes that there are many Japans, that it is not the uniform culture that is so often portrayed by both Japanese and foreign researchers. For some time Japanese researchers have been interested in the effect of regional climate and dietary variations on the incidence of disease (Oiso 1975). Educational and occupational differences are also important, and the continued occurrence of fox, badger, snake, and dog possession in specific geographical regions among less well educated people is one obvious example of this phenomenon (Yoshida 1967, 1972, 1984). A recent survey and cultural study of menopause in Japan used three subsamples: housewives, women employed in factories, and those running farms (Lock 1986a). Although little variation was found in the incidence of menopausal symptomatology (it was remarkably low in all three subsamples), both this study and Rosenberger's work presented in this volume graphically demonstrate how the social construction of menopause varies according to educational and occupational status. These recent studies of menopause raise further cautionary notes in the study of health and illness cross-culturally that lead us back to the problem of medicalization.

Menopause is a life-cycle transition that has become highly medicalized of late in the West. Important reasons for this are the aggressive marketing of estrogen replacement therapy and its adoption by gynecologists in their belief that it is an effective cure for symptomatology at menopause, which has been redefined in the medical literature as a "deficiency disease" (McCrea 1983). Physicians feel justified in their belief by the results they obtain when using estrogen replacement therapy with clinical populations in the West. Moreover, because they believe that biological changes at menopause are universal, they do not question the assumption that such treatment is also universally appropriate.

Lock's survey shows that Japanese women do not suffer to anything like the same degree from the symptoms that are commonly associated with menopause in the West, and recent research from other cultures has produced similar findings (Beyene 1986). This means that further comparative research is needed in order to unravel the various causal possibilities. Could these differences be accounted for by genetic, dietary, or climatic variation? Or are they differences due largely to the cultural interpretation of symptoms? Or does the fact that the problem is highly medicalized in the West and is much less so in Japan account for most of the difference? Or, and I am inclined to settle for this last possibility, are all three factors important? Whatever the answer, the findings raise for scrutiny assumptions made by medical professionals about the biological basis of menopause. These assumptions are being adopted at a rapid rate by Japanese gynecologists, although instead of citing the "hot flash" as the most frequently reported symptom, Japanese gynecologists resort to their early exposure to German medical knowledge and cite an imbalance of the autonomic nervous system as the biggest issue (Lock 1986a). We are beginning, therefore, to expose in the examination of menopause some of the same problems encountered by researchers working on depression.

The research of Rosenberger and Lock raises another crucial issue: the difference between actual symptomatology and the way in which ideas about events related to the body are subjected to shared cultural stereotypes of what should or is likely to happen. Rosenberger cites previous work to show that manipulation of the sick role is not uncommon in Japan, and her chapter here is an excellent study of how expectations about the experience of menopause are used in culturally appropriate ways by three samples of Japanese women. The meanings of menopause are interpreted in dramatically different styles in the three contexts and reflect regional differences in expected social roles as well as some of the changes that women's roles in general are undergoing in Japan today.

Symbolic use of the body is central to the Rosenberger and Lock chapters, but while Rosenberger focuses more on family dynamics and the changing roles of women, Lock surveys some of the historical and contemporary means of expressing protest and then analyzes the somatization of distress as one widely used form of dissent in Japan today (see also Ikemi and Ikemi 1982). She goes on to discuss the way in which somatized problems of women are managed in various clinical settings and makes extensive use of popular literature written by medical practitioners to illustrate the argument.

In common with all of the other contributors to this book, Lock demonstrates a great variation in the expression and management of medically related problems, albeit within certain ubiquitous cultural limitations. In the case of the medicalization of distress resulting from problems in which social precursors are heavily implicated, it is suggested that, while much contemporary medicalization acts to reduce psychosocial problems to the neutral terrain of the physical body, some of it may indeed serve to break down a little of the isolation that women experience in modern Japan. Hence medicalization may facilitate an ability to reinterpret the origins of distress as a social rather than a biological problem. We see some signs of this with the recent surge of interest in counseling and self-help groups, although naturally these groups also reflect shared Japanese values and do not function quite like their counterparts in the West (Lock n.d.).

The problems of women are not the only ones being medicalized. The press, popular medical literature, and government documents are rife with concern about "stress" and the reported increase of mental and physical illnesses thought to be associated with modernization, especially urbanization and the rise of the nuclear family. In addition to the numerous syndromes and neuroses associated exclusively with women, there are daily newspaper reports about "salary-man syndrome," "mal-adjustment-to-the-job syndrome," "school-refusal syndrome," parent abuse by children, bullying in school, and so on. Some authors write about the "pathological family" (Higuchi 1980).

What needs careful investigation is how these problems are used by people in power in both government and medical settings and by the media for their own ends. The statistics published on, for example, school-refusal syndrome show that the problem, although it clearly exists and is perhaps on the increase, is nevertheless still much smaller than anything that would cause ripples in North America (Monbushō 1983). The touting of glib articles on the latest syndrome has become part of the internal cultural debate *(nihonjinron)* on where the nation is heading and which values should be cultivated for success in the postindustrial age (Lock n.d.). Certainly many people are suffering both psychologi-cally and physically as a result of the enormous pressure imposed upon them by the stringent requirements of the Japanese labor and educa-tional system. Certainly many women, because of discrimination in employment and culturally inscribed values about the continued neces-sity of total dedication to maternal nurturance in an era of small families, are suffering from the opposite problem: a diminished social role. How-ever, with some notable exceptions (Yuzawa 1980) very little work has yet been done to distinguish the causes and incidence of genuine modern malaise from the poorly authenticated allegations of social disintegration that are perpetrated by partisan and powerful groups. It is disheartening that virtually without exception official and popular literature places the blame for all kinds of suffering firmly back onto the modern Japanese family, the "thinness" of its relationships and its lack of moral and tena-cious fiber (Lock 1986b; Iino 1980; Sasaki 1983; Monbushō 1983). The larger social contradictions and impasses, many of which are raised in this volume and are perhaps expressed most poignantly in Kiefer's discussion of the plight of the elderly and their female caretakers, remain relatively unquestioned and unexamined.

There is a call by the present Japanese government for a return to more traditional values, and in particular for a cultivation of something equivalent to the *ie,* the traditional Japanese household, where the young, the chronically sick, and the elderly would be fully taken care of. This is part of a plan for the "Japanese Welfare State" (McCormack 1986) and designed to avoid some of the pitfalls of what has been labeled the "English Disease" (see Steslicke, this volume). The creation of a modern version of the *ie* would, of course, if effective, relieve the government of the financial burden of improving and installing a range of health-related facilities. On the other hand, with urbanization, the existence of the nuclear family (which is unlikely to be replaced by a traditional extended family once again, despite attempts to do so), and the increasing desire of many middle-class women to participate seriously in the work force, the creation of a modern *ie* seems unrealistic. The absorption of the social side effects of urbanization, economic expansion, and technological progress by the family, in particular by an employed housewife living in an urban, nuclear household, is totally unrealistic. One cannot have one's tofu and eat it too. It remains to be seen how Japan will deal with the impasse it now seems to have reached after a period of incredibly rapid social change. I agree with Long in that I do not foresee a convergence with Western models for managing the problems of the modern world. On the contrary, I think that Japan is bent on creating its own specific, contextually relevant answers to these problems and that it will, therefore, continue to provide us with a rich source for the contrasting analysis of problems of all kinds, including those related to health and illness.

The essays that follow are designed to offer insights into several specific theoretical issues. They demonstrate, first, the importance of grounding studies of the body, health, and illness in rich empirical data and of analyzing that data from the perspective of each one of the social sciences. They are therefore an attempt to fill the lacuna that has arisen between "grand theory" such as that created, for example, by Foucault, Habermas, and Lacan, and highly descriptive microanalyses (Crews 1986). Second, the essays function, as does almost all social science done by both Japanese and Western scholars on Japan, to place similar studies done on the West in perspective and to show up some of the limitations of research designed without the benefits of cross-cultural insights. At the same time, some of the methods of dealing with problems of health and illness in Japan may provide insights for Western policymakers and practitioners. Third, the findings presented in these papers have important implications for developing countries, since they indicate some of the problems that are likely to arise in situations of rapid social change. Most especially they illustrate how biomedicine, when it is exported, does not simply alight in a vacuum and that it must be integrated into already existing beliefs and practices. The essays also illustrate some of the paradoxical outcomes that arise as the result of the application of modern medical technology.

In conclusion, it must be noted that it is unfortunate that no contributions to this volume have been made by Japanese researchers, an unavoidable result of the exigencies of current funding in the social sciences. We look forward to being involved with our Japanese colleagues in future conferences and publications. In the meantime, we welcome their comments and criticisms and hope that this volume may provide some incentive for a pooling of our knowledge and methodological inclinations.

References

Abe, M. 1985. Japan's clinic physicians and their behavior. *Social Science and Medicine* 20:335–340.

Abrams, H. K. 1979. Together with the farmers. *Agricultural Medicine and Rural Health* 4:35–41.

Armstrong, D. 1983. *Political anatomy of the body.* Cambridge: Cambridge Univ. Press.

Beardsley, R. K., J. W. Hall, and R. E. Ward. 1959. *Village Japan.* Chicago: Univ. of Chicago Press.

Beeman, W. O. 1985. Dimensions of dysphoria. In *Culture and depression,* ed. A. Kleinman and B. Good. Berkeley and Los Angeles, Univ. of California Press.

Beyene, Y. 1986. Cultural significance and physiological manifestations of menopause. *Culture, Medicine and Psychiatry* 10:47–71.

Bourdieu, P. 1977. *Outline of a theory of practice.* Trans. Richard Nice. Cambridge: Cambridge Univ. Press.

Campbell, J. C. 1984. Problems, solutions, non-solutions, and free medical care for the elderly in Japan. *Pacific Affairs* 57:53–64.

Campbell, R. 1984. Nursing homes and long-term care in Japan. *Pacific Affairs* 57:78–89.

Caudill, W. 1962. Patterns of emotion in modern Japan. In *Japanese culture*, ed. R. J. Smith and R. K. Beardsley. Chicago: Aldine.

———. 1976. Everyday health and illness in Japan and America. In *Asian medical systems*, ed. C. Leslie. Berkeley and Los Angeles: Univ. of California Press.

Caudill, W., and T. Doi. 1963. Inter-relations of psychiatry, culture and emotion in Japan. In *Man's image in medicine and anthropology*, ed. I. Galdston. New York: International Univ. Press.

Cohen, J., S. L. Syme, C. D. Jenkins, A. Kagan, and S. V. Zyzanski. 1979. Cultural context of Type A behavior and risk for CHD. *Journal of Behavioral Medicine* 2:375–384.

Coleman, S. 1983. *Family planning in Japanese society*. Princeton: Princeton Univ. Press.

Comaroff, J. 1985. *Body of power, spirit of resistance*. Chicago: Univ. of Chicago Press.

Crews, F. 1986. The house of grand theory. *New York Review of Books* 33:36–41.

Davis, W. 1980. *Dojo*. Stanford: Stanford Univ. Press.

DeVos, G. 1973. *Socialization for achievement*. Berkeley and Los Angeles: Univ. of California Press.

DeVos, G., and H. Wagatsuma. 1959. Psychocultural significance of concern over death and illness among rural Japanese. *International Journal of Social Psychiatry* 5:5–19.

Doi, T. 1973. *The anatomy of dependence*. Tokyo: Kodansha.

———. 1986. *The anatomy of self*. Tokyo: Kodansha.

Douglas, M. 1970. *Natural symbols*. London: Barrie and Rockliff.

Embree, J. F. 1939. *Suye Mura*. Chicago: Univ. of Chicago Press.

Feldman, E. 1985. Medical ethics the Japanese way. *Hastings Center Report* 15:21–30.

Foucault, M. 1973. *The birth of the clinic*. London: Tavistock.

———. 1979. *Discipline and punish*. New York: Random House.

Freidson, E. 1970. *Profession of medicine*. New York: Dodd, Mead, and Co.

Fukutake, T. 1980. *Japanese rural society*. Tokyo: Univ. of Tokyo Press.

Goldsmith, S. 1984. Hospitals and the elderly in Japan. *Pacific Affairs* 57:74–77.

Hahn, R. A., and A. D. Gaines. 1985. *Physicians of western society*. Boston: D. Reidel.

Helman, C. G. 1978. "Feed a cold, starve a fever." *Culture, Medicine and Psychiatry* 2:107–137.

Higuchi, K. 1980. Changing family relationships. *Japan Echo* 7:86–93.

Honda, Y. 1983. DSM-III in Japan. In *International perspectives on DSM-III*, ed. R. L. Spitzer, J. B. W. Williams, and A. E. Skodol. Washington, D.C.: American Psychiatric Association.

Iga, M. 1986. *The thorn in the chrysanthemum.* Berkeley and Los Angeles: Univ. of California Press.

Iga, M. et al. 1978. Suicide in Japan. Special issue, Social science and medicine in Japan. *Social Science and Medicine* 12:507–516.

Iino, S. 1980. *Tōkōkyohi no kokufukuhō* (Methods for resolving school refusal). Tokyo: Bunrishoin.

Ikegami, N. 1980. Growth of psychiatric beds in Japan. *Social Science and Medicine* 14:561–570.

Ikemi, Y., and A. Ikemi. 1982. Some psychosomatic disorders in Japan in a cultural perspective. *Psychotherapy and Psychosomatics* 38:231–238.

Ikemi, Y., et al. 1980. Psychosomatic mechanism under social changes in Japan. In *Biopsychosocial health,* ed. S. B. Day, F. Lolas, and M. Kusinitz. New York: A monograph publication in health communications and biopsychosocial health of the International Foundation for Biosocial Development and Human Health.

Illich, I. D. 1976. *Medical nemesis.* New York: Pantheon.

Katon, W., R. Ries, and A. Kleinman. 1984. The prevalence of somatization in primary care. *Comprehensive Psychiatry* 25 (2): 208–215.

Kleinman, A. M. 1979. *Patients and healers in the context of culture.* Berkeley and Los Angeles: Univ. of California Press.

Lebra, T. 1974. Interactional perspective on suffering and curing in a Japanese cult. *International Journal of Social Psychiatry* 20:281–286.

———. 1976a. *Japanese patterns of behavior.* Honolulu: Univ. of Hawaii Press.

———. 1976b. Taking the role of the supernatural "other." In *Culture-bound syndromes, ethnopsychiatry and alternate therapies,* ed. W. P. Lebra. Honolulu: Univ. of Hawaii Press, an East-West Center Book.

———. 1982. Self-reconstruction in Japanese religious psychotherapy. In *Cultural conceptions of mental health and therapy,* ed. A. J. Marsella and G. M. White. Boston: D. Reidel.

Leslie, C. 1976. *Asian medical systems.* Berkeley and Los Angeles: Univ. of California Press.

Lock, M. 1980. *East Asian medicine in urban Japan.* Berkeley and Los Angeles: Univ. of California Press.

———. 1982a. The organization and practice of East Asian medicine in Japan. *Social Science and Medicine* 14B:245–253.

———. 1982b. Popular conceptions of mental health in Japan. In *Cultural conceptions of mental health and therapy,* ed. A. J. Marsella and G. M. White. Boston: D. Reidel.

———. 1984a. East Asian medicine and health care for the Japanese elderly. *Pacific Affairs* 57 (1): 65–73.

———. 1984b. Licorice in leviathan. *Culture, Medicine and Psychiatry* 8:121–139.

————. 1986a. Ambiguities of aging. *Culture, Medicine and Psychiatry* 10:23–46.

————. 1986b. Plea for acceptance. *Social Science and Medicine* 23:99–112.

————. n.d. Faltering discipline and the ailing family in Japan. In *Paths of Asian medical knowledge,* ed. A. Young. Boston: D. Reidel. Forthcoming.

Long. S. O. 1980. Fame, fortune, and friends. Ph.D. diss. University of Illinois, Urbana.

————. 1984. The sociocultural context of nursing in Japan. *Culture, Medicine and Psychiatry* 8:141–164.

————. 1986. Roles, careers and femininity in biomedicine. *Social Science and Medicine* 22:81–90.

Long, S. O., and B. Long. 1982. Curable cancers and fatal ulcers. *Social Science and Medicine* 16:2101–2108.

McCormack, G. 1986. Beyond economism. In *Democracy in Contemporary Japan,* ed. G. McCormack and Y. Sugimoto. Sydney: Hale and Iremongo.

McCrea, F. 1983. The politics of menopause. *Social Problems* 31:111–123.

McKean, M. A. 1981. *Environmental protest and citizen politics in Japan.* Berkeley and Los Angeles: Univ. of California Press.

McKeown, T. 1976. *The modern rise of population.* New York: Academic Press.

Marmot, M., and S. L. Syme. 1976. Acculturation and coronary heart disease in Japanese-Americans. *American Journal of Epidemiology* 104:225–247.

Marsella, A. J. 1980. Depression experience and disorder across cultures. In *Handbook of cross-cultural psychology.* Vol. 6, *Psychopathology,* ed. H. Triandis and J. Draguns. Rockleigh, N.J.: Allyn and Bacon.

Marsella, A. J. et al. 1985. Cross-cultural studies of depressive disorders. In *Culture and depression,* ed. A. Kleinman and B. Good. Berkeley and Los Angeles: Univ. of California Press.

Martin, A. 1939. The bath in Japan. *Ciba Symposium* 1:156–162.

Miyasaka, T. 1971. An evaluation of a ten-year demonstration project in community health in a rural area in Japan. *Social Science and Medicine* 5:425–440.

Monbushō. 1983. *Tōkōkyohi mondai o chūshin ni* (Paying attention to the school refusal problem). Tokyo.

Munakata, T. 1986. Social-cultural background of the mental health system in Japan. *Culture, Medicine and Psychiatry* 10:351–356.

Nakane, C. 1970. *Japanese society.* Berkeley and Los Angeles: Univ. of California Press.

Navarro, V. 1976. *Medicine under capitalism.* New York: Prodist.

Niki, R. 1985. The wide distribution of CT scanners in Japan. *Social Science and Medicine* 21:1131–1137.

Nikkei Medical. 1981. Chōsa: daiisen rinshōi no kampōyaku shiyō jōkyō (A survey of the use of *kampōyaku* by clinicians). 10:28–31.

Nishirai, T. 1983. *For the sake of the people.* JOICFP Document Series 9. Tokyo: Japanese Organization for International Cooperation in Family Planning.

Norbeck, E. 1954. *Takashima.* Salt Lake City: Univ. of Utah Press.

Ohara, K. 1973. The socio-cultural approach for the manic-depressive psychosis. *Psychiatrica et Neurologica Japonica* 75:263–273.

Ohnuki-Tierney, E. 1984. *Illness and culture in contemporary Japan.* Cambridge: Cambridge Univ. Press.

Oiso, T. 1975. Incidence of stomach cancer and its relation to dietary habits and nutrition in Japan between 1900 and 1975. *Cancer Research* 35:3254–3258.

Okino, T. 1978. Health and social factors in Japan. Special issue, Social science and medicine in Japan. *Social Science and Medicine* 12:459–468.

Reich, M. 1984. Troubles, issues and politics in Japan. In *Institutions for changing Japanese society,* ed. G. DeVos. Research Papers and Policy Issues. Berkeley: Institute of East Asian Studies, Univ. of California.

Reynolds, D. K. 1976. *Morita psychotherapy.* Berkeley and Los Angeles: Univ. of California Press.

———. 1980. *The quiet therapies.* Honolulu: Univ. of Hawaii Press.

———. 1981. Naikan therapy. In *Handbook of innovative psychotherapies,* ed. R. Corsini. New York: Wiley.

Sasaki, H. 1983. *Kokoro no kenkō sōdanshitsu* (Consultations for mental health). Tokyo: Asahi Shimbunsha.

Scotch, N. 1963. Sociocultural factors in the epidemiology of Zulu hypertension. *American Journal of Public Health* 53:1203–1213.

Shinfuku, N. et al. 1973. Changing clinical pictures of depression. *Psychological Medicine* 15:955–965.

Smith, R. J. 1974. *Ancestor worship in contemporary Japan.* Stanford: Stanford Univ. Press.

———. 1978. *Kurusu.* Stanford: Stanford Univ. Press.

Smith, T. C. 1977. *Nakahara.* Stanford: Stanford Univ. Press.

Steslicke, W. 1982a. Development of health insurance policy in Japan. *Journal of Health Politics, Policy and the Law* 7:197–226.

———. 1982b. Medical care for Japan's aging population. *Pacific Affairs* 57:45–52.

———. 1982c. National health policy in Japan. *Bulletin of the Institute for Public Health* 31:1–35.

Tanaka-Matsumi, J. 1979. Taijin kyufushō. *Culture, Medicine and Psychiatry* 3:231–245.

Tanaka-Matsumi, J., and A. J. Marsella. 1976. Cross-cultural variations in the phenomenological experience of depression. *Journal of Cross-Cultural Psychology* 7:379-396.

Tatara, M. 1982. Psychoanalytic psychotherapy in Japan. *Journal of the American Academy of Psychoanalysis* 10:225-239.

Tsunoda, T. 1979. Difference in the mechanism of emotion in Japanese and Westerner. *Psychotherapy and Psychosomatics* 31:367-372.

Turner, B. 1984. *The body and society.* Oxford: Basil Blackwell.

Worsley, P. 1982. Non-western medical systems. *Annual Review of Anthropology* 11:315-348.

Yamamoto, M. 1978. A review of development in social sciences in relation to health and medical care in Japan. *Social Science and Medicine* 12:443-449.

Yamamoto, M., and J. Ohmura. 1975. The health and medical system in Japan. *Inquiry,* supplement to vol. 12:42-50.

Yoshida, T. 1967. Mystical retribution, spirit possession, and social structure in a Japanese village. *Ethnology* 6:237-262.

————. 1972. *Nihon no tsukimono* (Japanese possession spirits). Tokyo: Chūkōshinsho.

————. 1984. Spirit possession and village conflict. In *Conflict in Japan,* ed. E. S. Krauss, T. P. Rohlen, and P. G. Steinhoff. Honolulu: Univ. of Hawaii Press.

Yoshida, Y., and K. Yoshida. 1976. The high rate of appendectomy in Japan. *Medical Care* 14:950-957.

Yoshimita, T., M. Kawano, and I. Takayama. 1971. Masked depression in the department of internal medicine. *Journal of the Japanese Psychosomatic Society* 11:48.

Yuzawa, Y. 1980. Nihon no katei wa honto ni yande iru· no ka (Is the Japanese family really in trouble?). *Asahi Jaanaru.*

Zola, I. K. 1978. Medicine as an institution of social control. In *The cultural crisis of modern medicine,* ed. J. Ehrenreich. New York: Monthly Review Press.

The Japanese State of Health: A Political-Economic Perspective

WILLIAM E. STESLICKE

The Postwar "Health Miracle"

When compared with conditions at the end of World War II, the generally high standard of living enjoyed by contemporary Japanese seems amazing.[1] Indeed, the recovery from the devastation of defeat and the subsequent rapid growth in the production of goods and services are often referred to as Japan's "economic miracle." The international attention and acclaim that Japan's economic recovery and growth have received have, in fact, tended to overshadow other postwar Japanese accomplishments. Yet, to borrow a metaphor, a virtual "health miracle" has also taken place in postwar Japan. In terms of most commonly accepted indicators, the Japanese state of health at the beginning of the 1980s was among the highest in the world. In 1945 the estimated life expectancy at birth for Japanese males was 23.9 years and for females 37.5 years. By 1984 the average life expectancy for males had increased to 74.54 years and for females to 80.18 years (table 1). These figures were the highest in the world.

Japan's economic and health "miracles" are not unrelated. As pointed out in the recent World Health Organization study, "Countries with a high gross national product have a low infant mortality rate and a high life expectancy, the opposite being the case for countries with a low GNP" (WHO 1981, 21–22). Although a number of other factors contribute to the state of health in various nations, clearly economic development provides the capacity for bringing other important factors into play. Still, it would be wrong to conclude that the relationship is simple and unilinear (Abel-Smith 1976, 138–197; Renaud 1975, 559–571). Improved health status and effective public health and medical care programs contribute to economic development, but economic development

Table 1. Average Life Expectancy at Birth: Japan and Other Nations

Country	Men	Country	Women
Japan	74.54	Japan	80.18
Iceland	73.91	Sweden	79.61
Sweden	73.62	Iceland	79.45
Holland	72.70	Norway	79.41
Norway	72.64	Holland	79.40
United States	71.60	France	78.85
England and Wales	71.09	United States	78.80
France	70.73	England and Wales	77.11
Federal Republic of Germany	70.46	Federal Republic of Germany	77.09

Source: Kōsei Tōkei Kyōkai (1985, 79).
Note: Figures for Japan, 1984; Iceland, 1981–1982; Sweden, 1983; Holland, 1982; Norway, 1981–1982; United States, 1983; England, 1980–1982; France, 1982; Federal Republic of Germany, 1981–1983.

also gives rise to new health hazards. If the Japanese have enjoyed the benefits of economic development, the victims of Minamata disease, Yokkaichi asthma, "Itai-Itai" disease, and other ailments can testify to the pain that has accompanied the high-growth strategy of the postwar period. Admirers of the Japanese model tend to ignore this side of the balance sheet (Huddle and Reich 1975).

Neither "miracle," therefore, is without blemish. Nor is it possible to certify the intervention of a divine hand in the economic and health sectors. Much more apparent in both cases is the intervention of the Japanese state and its only too mortal agents. While a precise measurement of cause and effect is impossible, the evidence strongly supports the proposition that a Japanese version of the "developmental state" was an essential component of high economic growth.[2] The concept of a "developmental state" and the particular set of priorities adopted by its agents are also important to an appreciation of the state of health in contemporary Japan and the problems and issues of the present and foreseeable future (Steslicke 1982c). A brief review of the Japanese state of health as of 1980 in terms of some of the more widely used indicators is a necessary preface to further discussion.

The Japanese State *of* Health

To the extent that such things can be ascertained by national surveys, it appears that Japanese citizens place a very high priority on good health and medical care. Every three years since 1972 the Economic Planning Agency has conducted national surveys on living standards. These surveys utilize ten categories related to daily life: (1) education and culture, (2) employment and quality of working life, (3) family, (4) income and consumption, (5) justice and social welfare, (6) living environment, (7) medical care and health, (8) quality of community life, (9) security and protection of individuals, and (10) vacation and leisure. In response to the question, "Which areas are important to your life at present and in the future?" 35.3 percent of those selected for the 1981 survey indicated that medical care and health was their top priority. Roughly 84 percent included medical care and health among their top five priorities. Not only the mature and elderly, but all segments of the population placed a high priority on medical care and health (Economic Planning Agency 1981, 243).

Although it is difficult to assess the importance of attitudes on the actual distribution of health and illness in the population, the generally positive orientation to health and medical care in Japan is surely an important influence on the state of health as measured by the conventional objective indicators.[3] Certainly, attitudes have an important bearing on the more qualitative aspects of health and medical care (Caudill 1976). Also, widespread expectations of a long and healthy life must be taken into account by those who seek to establish and implement national priorities. Not only was life expectancy at birth the highest in the world as of 1980, so too was life expectancy at age sixty for both men (18.27 years) and women (21.96 years).[4] These expectations place new burdens on the health care system as well as on national resources in general. Given the imperatives of Japan's rapidly aging society and the leveling off of economic growth, it may prove impossible to improve or even maintain the comparatively high state of health (Ogawa 1982; Tominaga 1983). Whether the positive orientation toward health and medical care will be sustained remains to be seen.

One of two persons born in 1980 could expect to live to age eighty; however, in that same year 722,792 persons died. The fluctuation in the death rate per 1,000 persons between 1955 and 1980 was slight (from 7.8 to 6.2 per 1,000 persons). However, the age distribution changed markedly. In 1955, of 690,000 deaths, 17.3 percent were fourteen years of age or below; in 1980 this ratio dropped to 2.9 percent. A corresponding decrease in the mortality rate in the age fifteen to sixty-four category from 38.6 percent to 27.5 percent was also recorded. By 1980, 69.6 percent of the deaths were among persons of sixty-five years or older, as compared with 44.1 percent in 1955. The changing distribution reflects the demographic change that has taken place and the sharp decrease in infant mortality as well as in tuberculosis-related deaths in the age category fifteen to sixty-four.

In causes of death, the increase is quite remarkable in so-called adult diseases, particularly cancer, heart disease, and cirrhosis of the liver. Between 1960 and 1980, cerebrovascular and hypertensive disease as causes of death increased by 8.1 percent and 5.3 percent, respectively, but cancer increased by 72.4 percent, heart disease by 80.5 percent, and cirrhosis of the liver by 81.6 percent. The increase in the latter was especially sharp in the forty to fifty age category. There was a decrease in tuberculosis, gastroenteritis, gastric ulcer, nephritis, and pneumonia as causes of death over the same period. Table 2 shows the change in incidence of the causes of death between 1960 and 1980. Although the top three held fast during that period, the relative increase in cancer and heart disease has aroused considerable concern. In table 3, the leading causes of death in Japan in 1980 are compared with figures from four other major industrial nations. It is interesting that Japan compares quite favorably with these nations in terms of motor vehicle and other accidental deaths. Between 1960 and 1980, the rate per 100,000 of accidental deaths decreased from 41.7 in 1960 and 42.5 in 1970 to 13.7 in 1980. This means about 30,000 accidental deaths a year at present, of which over 13,000 are motor vehicle or traffic related. It has been estimated that in the postwar era one of every ten Japanese has been injured in a traffic accident. Obviously, given the spectacular increase in automobiles in recent times, the problem is chronic (Kubota 1980; Japan Institute of Labor 1982).

Work-related deaths and injuries are similarly chronic. In 1980, 3,009 persons were killed and 336,000 persons injured at work. The trend in work-related fatalities between 1965 and 1980 is shown in table 4. As indicated, there has been a steady decline since 1965, especially in the construction and manufacturing industries and, as a consequence of the reduction in scale of those industries, a corresponding decline in mining and forestry fatalities and injuries.

Finally, note should be taken of suicide as a cause of death (21.6 per 100,000 population in 1960, 15.3 in 1970, and 17.7 in 1980). A great deal has been written about the relatively high rate of suicide in contemporary Japan (see, for example, Iga et al. 1978). What is not widely

Table 2. Leading Causes of Death in Japan, 1960–1980

Rank	1960	1970	1980
1	Cerebrovascular disease (160.7)	Cerebrovascular disease (175.8)	Cerebrovascular disease (139.7)
2	Cancer (100.4)	Cancer (116.3)	Cancer (139.2)
3	Heart disease (73.2)	Heart disease (86.7)	Heart disease (106.3)
4	Senility (58.0)	Accidents (42.5)	Pneumonia (33.8)
5	Pneumonia (49.3)	Senility (38.1)	Senility (27.7)
6	Accidents (41.7)	Pneumonia (34.1)	Hypertensive disease (25.1)
7	Tuberculosis (34.2)	Hypertensive disease (17.7)	Suicides (17.7)
8	Suicides (21.6)	Tuberculosis (15.4)	Cirrhosis of the liver (14.2)
9	Gastro-enteritis (21.6)	Suicides (15.3)	Accidents (13.7)
10	Infant mortality (18.5)	Cirrhosis of the liver (12.5)	Nephritis (8.8)

Source: Economic Planning Agency, Govt. of Japan (1981, 105).
Note: Figures in parentheses indicate death rate per 100,000 population.

known, however, is the increased incidence among middle-aged males since the late 1960s. In the 1950s and 1960s, the age distribution of suicides described an "N" curve, with one peak at the twenty to twenty-four age group, the other at the high end of the age scale, with the thirty-five to forty-four age group providing the valley. The postwar high in the suicide rate (25.7 persons per 100,000) was reached in 1958. The rate then declined to a postwar low of 14.2 per 100,000 in 1967. There has been a gradual increase since then, mainly in the former valley of middle-aged males—thus changing the shape of the "N" curve. According to National Police Agency data for 1980 related to motives for suicide, within the age forty to forty-nine category, 35.1 percent apparently

Table 3. Leading Causes of Death in Five Industrial Nations

Cause of death	Japan (1980)	U.S.A. (1977)	U.K. (1977)	France (1976)	West Germany (1978)
Heart disease	106.3	327.2	379.1	200.2	335.1
Cancer	139.2	178.7	254.9	225.4	252.9
Cerebrovascular disease	139.7	84.1	149.3	141.0	166.0
Cirrhosis of the liver	14.2	14.3	3.7	32.9	27.6
Motor vehicle accidents	10.1	22.9	11.9	23.3	23.1
Other accidents	15.0	24.8	17.4	48.6	26.1
Suicides	17.7	13.3	8.0	15.8	22.2
Total causes	622.0	877.9	1,172.5	1,051.6	1,179.3

Source: Economic Planning Agency, Govt. of Japan (1981, 107).
Note: Unit: number of deaths per 100,000 persons.

Table 4. Work-Related Fatalities in Japan, 1965–1980

Year \ Industry types	Construction	Manufacture	Transportation	Minery	Forestry	Others	Total
(Actual number)	person	person	person	person	person	person	person
1965	2,251	1,161	674	960	319	681	6,045
1970	2,430	1,400	674	474	248	822	6,048
1975	1,582	856	375	224	153	535	3,725
1976	1,451	669	371	170	136	548	3,345
1977	1,464	709	344	180	131	474	3,302
1978	1,583	650	303	135	135	520	3,326
1979	1,404	594	331	149	115	484	3,077
1980	1,374	589	313	105	117	511	3,009
(Percentage)	%	%	%	%	%	%	%
1965	37.2	19.2	11.1	15.9	5.3	11.3	100.0
1970	40.2	23.2	11.1	7.8	4.1	13.6	100.0
1975	42.5	23.0	10.1	6.0	4.1	14.3	100.0
1980	45.6	19.6	10.4	3.5	3.9	17.0	100.0
(Change in percentage)	%	%	%	%	%	%	%
1970/1965	8.0	20.6	0.0	Δ50.6	Δ22.3	20.7	0.0
1975/1970	Δ34.9	Δ38.9	Δ44.4	Δ52.7	Δ38.3	Δ34.9	Δ38.4
1980/1975	Δ13.1	Δ31.2	Δ16.5	Δ53.1	Δ23.5	Δ 4.5	Δ19.2

Source: Economic Planning Agency, Govt. of Japan (1981, 117).

suffered from disease, but 20.4 percent were apparently troubled by economic problems (table 5).

Before shifting the focus of this review from mainly mortality-related statistics to an examination of morbidity indicators, it should once again be emphasized that definitive description of the national state of health is not the objective here.[5] Rather, the more limited goal is to present such information as is readily available in support of the general impression that the state of health in Japan has a high international ranking. The most important source of data is the annual National Health Survey (Kokumin Kenkō Chōsa) conducted since 1953 by the Ministry of Health and Welfare (Kōseishō). In 1980 some 54,000 persons from 16,000 households selected as a stratified random sample were interviewed between September 15 and 17 in order to estimate the extent of injury, disease, and medical treatment in Japan. Some of the major findings follow.

Of the total number of households included in the sample, 25.9 percent reported one or more injured or diseased members (up from 25.8 percent in 1979) and 10.0 percent of those individuals interviewed reported personal injury or disease (also 10.0 percent in 1979). In terms of the morbidity or prevalence rate, estimated at 110.4 per 1,000 persons, it seems that one in every 9.1 Japanese was injured or ill in 1980. This figure has remained relatively stable for the past several years. As indicated in table 6, diseases of the circulatory system had the highest rate at 36.6. Within that category, the rate of hypertensive disease was 24.1 per 1,000 persons. Diseases of the respiratory system (15.5) and diseases of the digestive system (14.4) were the next two highest categories reported.

Table 7 shows morbidity rates by disease and age bracket. Note that

Table 5. Motive for Suicide in Japan, 1980

	Suffering from Diseases	Alcoholism– Mental Disorder	Home- Related Problems	Work- Related Problems	Economic Problems	Other
All ages (male and female)	44.3%	16.6%	10.6%	4.4%	8.6%	15.5%
Ages 40–49 (male)	35.1%	15.1%	10.2%	7.3%	20.4%	11.9%

Source: Economic Planning Agency, Govt. of Japan (1981, 109).

Table 6. Yearly Change in Prevalence Rates by Category per 1,000 Persons

Disease \ Year	1955	1965	1970	1975	1976	1977	1978	1979	1980
Infectious and parasitic diseases	7.7	4.4	3.7	2.5	3.7	3.6	2.8	2.9	2.5
Neoplasms	0.5	0.9	0.8	0.9	0.8	0.9	0.9	0.8	0.9
Endocrine, nutritional and metabolic diseases, and immunity disorders	0.7	1.2	2.0	2.6	3.1	3.5	3.3	4.9	5.4
Diseases of the blood and blood-forming organs	0.2	0.5	0.7	0.8	0.8	0.8	0.8	0.9	0.8
Mental disorders	0.4	1.1	1.1	0.9	1.1	1.0	1.0	1.2	0.9
Diseases of the nervous system and sense organs	4.8	7.9	11.2	10.4	12.0	9.8	9.3	5.4	5.8
Diseases of the circulatory system	3.3	11.9	21.6	23.3	28.7	30.1	26.6	31.3	36.6
Hypertensive diseases	1.3	8.0	14.6	15.6	19.5	20.1	17.5	20.8	24.1
Diseases of the respiratory system	5.5	8.2	14.4	30.8	26.3	25.8	25.5	17.9	15.5
Acute nasopharingitis	—	—	9.6	25.3	20.9	20.2	20.0	13.5	9.6
Diseases of the digestive system	6.5	13.8	17.9	15.4	16.2	16.4	16.5	15.9	14.4
Diseases of dental and dental sustentacular tissue	1.9	5.0	6.9	3.8	3.8	3.9	3.9	3.4	3.4
Diseases of the genitourinary system	0.8	1.6	1.8	2.3	2.4	2.6	2.9	2.4	2.4
Complications of pregnancy, childbirth, and the puerperium	0.2	0.2	0.1	0.1	0.2	0.1	0.1	0.2	0.2
Diseases of the skin and subcutaneous tissue	2.0	2.1	3.2	3.5	3.7	3.1	2.7	3.0	3.3
Diseases of the musculoskeletal system and connective tissue	1.5	3.6	5.6	6.3	6.5	7.6	7.3	11.9	10.7
Congenital anomalies	0.1	0.2	0.3	0.2	0.2	0.3	0.1	0.2	0.3
Certain conditions originating in the perinatal period	0.0	0.1	—	0.0	0.0	0.0	0.0	—	0.0
Symptoms, signs, and ill-defined conditions	1.0	1.2	2.5	2.5	1.9	2.4	2.4	2.7	2.2
Injury and poisoning	2.3	4.2	6.2	7.4	8.8	7.4	8.5	7.6	8.5
Treatment with dental prosthetic device	0.4	0.5	0.6	0.1	0.1	0.2	0.1	0.2	0.0
Total	37.9	63.6	93.6	109.9	116.4	115.7	110.9	109.4	110.4

Source: Ministry of Health and Welfare (1981b, 5).
Note: The 9th International classification for disease, injury, and cause of death has been adopted since 1979. For this reason the names of diseases and classifications may not necessarily coincide with those prior to 1978.

Table 7. Prevalence Rates by Disease and Age Bracket

Disease	Total	0–4	5–14
Infectious and parasitic diseases	2.5	4.6	2.6
Neoplasms	0.9	0.5	0.2
Endocrine, nutritional and metabolic diseases, and immunity disorders	5.4	—	—
Diseases of the blood and blood-forming organs	0.8	—	—
Mental disorders	0.9	—	—
Diseases of the nervous system and sense organs	5.8	4.8	4.1
Diseases of the circulatory system	36.6	0.5	0.3
Hypertensive diseases	24.1	—	—
Diseases of the respiratory system	15.5	48.6	24.9
Acute nasopharingitis	9.6	42.9	13.5
Diseases of the digestive system	14.4	3.8	5.1
Diseases of dental and dental sustentacular tissue	3.4	1.9	4.1
Diseases of the genitourinary system	2.4	—	0.9
Complications of pregnancy, childbirth, and the puerperium	0.2	—	—
Diseases of the skin and subcutaneous tissue	3.3	9.7	4.7
Diseases of the musculoskeletal system and connective tissue	10.7	—	0.8
Congenital anomalies	0.3	0.8	0.4
Certain conditions originating in the perinatal period	0.0	0.3	—
Symptoms, signs, and ill-defined conditions	2.2	1.6	1.9
Injury and poisoning	8.5	13.3	10.1
Treatment with dental prosthetic device	0.0	—	—
Total	110.4	87.4	56.0

Source: Ministry of Health and Welfare (1981a, 6).

Categories per 1,000 Persons

15–24	25–34	35–44	45–54	55–64	65–74	75 and above	70 and above
0.3	2.1	1.7	3.3	2.5	5.3	2.9	3.8
0.1	0.1	0.6	2.2	0.4	3.2	5.3	4.4
0.7	1.8	4.0	5.6	14.1	23.4	14.1	19.3
0.1	0.2	0.9	1.0	1.9	2.9	2.9	2.2
0.9	1.5	1.0	1.4	0.8	1.2	0.6	1.6
1.7	2.4	3.8	4.2	10.4	18.4	28.8	23.7
0.7	2.9	13.2	40.4	106.7	173.7	241.9	224.2
0.1	0.6	9.2	30.3	70.8	113.5	150.1	141.5
7.1	10.1	8.8	8.3	12.0	18.1	21.2	20.2
5.1	7.4	5.5	4.1	2.6	6.7	9.4	8.2
5.6	7.9	16.4	24.0	30.5	29.5	27.1	30.9
2.2	3.2	4.2	4.0	3.7	3.5	0.6	1.6
1.3	2.3	2.7	3.0	4.4	3.2	8.2	5.7
0.4	0.6	0.2	—	—	—	—	—
2.5	2.3	2.7	1.5	3.1	2.0	5.3	3.8
1.4	2.5	7.0	12.7	30.9	42.7	53.6	54.0
0.1	—	0.2	—	0.6	0.6	1.2	0.9
—	—	—	—	—	—	—	—
1.2	1.4	1.8	3.3	1.5	2.0	14.1	8.5
5.9	5.2	9.2	8.0	10.2	9.6	10.0	10.4
—	0.1	—	—	—	—	—	—
30.2	43.4	74.3	121.8	229.9	336.0	437.3	413.6

the general rate of 87.4 in the zero to four age group tapers off to a low of 30.2 in the fifteen to twenty-four age group, and then gradually increases to 437.3 in the seventy-five and above bracket. Persons under thirty-five years old reported the highest rate for diseases of the respiratory system; those between thirty-five and forty-four, digestive disorders; and persons forty-five and above, diseases of the circulatory system. The overall morbidity rate was higher for females (117.8) than for males (102.6) and higher in large cities (121.7) than in smaller communities, where the morbidity rates ranged from 103.4 to 112.0. Males reported the highest rates for injury and poisoning and females reported the highest rates for diseases of the circulatory system, musculoskeletal system and connective tissue, nervous system, and sense organs.

It is worth noting that, while seven of every ten persons reported that they were in good health, only 1.3 percent indicated that they had received no medical treatment during the year of the survey. Of those receiving some sort of treatment, 87.5 percent went to hospitals or clinics, 8.8 percent purchased drugs at pharmacies, and 1.4 percent relied on massage, acupuncture, moxibustion, and judo corrective exercises. Of the total, over 40 percent reported taking at least one type of medication during the month before the survey.

Concluding this review of the Japanese state of health, it should be noted that the majority of those included in the 1980 survey (61.9 percent) reported that they had not been confined to bed during the survey year, and 30.5 percent reported bed stays of from one to ten days. As might be expected, the older age groups reported more and longer bed stays, but the majority of persons in all age categories, including those of years seventy-five and older, reported no bed stays. Nevertheless, the institutionalization rate for the population sixty-five and older is quite high, having increased from 0.9 percent in 1955 to 5.6 percent in 1980 (Ikegami 1982, 2001). How to cope with this and other health and medical care problems related to the rapid aging of the population is an item high on the agenda for the health policymakers in contemporary Japan.

The Japanese State *in* Health

In the post–World War II era, public health and welfare activities of the Japanese "developmental state" have had an explicit constitutional basis. According to Article 25 of the Japanese constitution (adopted in 1947), all citizens are guaranteed "the right to maintain the minimum standards of wholesome and cultured living." Article 25 also provides that "in all spheres of life, the state shall use its endeavors for the promotion and extension of social welfare and security, and of public health." During the 1950s and 1960s, the Japanese state appeared reluctant to fill this constitutional prescription and within the club of advanced industrial and capitalist nations was generally perceived as a "welfare laggard" (Bennett and Levine 1976, 442). By the end of the 1970s, however, both the image and the reality of the Japanese welfare state changed considerably. Not only was the constitutional prescription being filled, but some critics claimed that Japan had become a "welfare superstate." Others warned of the dangers of incipient "English Disease." A close examination of the role of the Japanese state in the health sector fails to confirm the diagnosis—nor does it support either the "laggard" or the "superstate" assessment.

To understand the contemporary situation, it is important to know something about the historical context. As noted earlier, the achievements of the Japanese state in the health sector since 1945 seem substantial. Consider, for example, the following assessment of the health and welfare administration made by officials of the Public Health and Welfare Section, General Headquarters, Supreme Commander for the Allied Powers:

> During the war increased industrialization and urbanization in the four main islands of Japan, plus the dominance of the military aims over all social welfare activities, had a pronounced influence on public health and welfare administration. Pressure of militarism brought greater emphasis on such emergency requirements as a rapid turn out of medical students, nurses and dentists. It also resulted in the cessation of many public health activities of benefit to the civilian population. The conversion of many factories, engaged in the manufacture of medical and sanitary supplies and equipment, to war material production, plus the lack of adequate professional people to serve the civilian population, resulted in a complete breakdown of all public health and welfare functions. From the national to the lowest level the entire administration of public health and welfare activities became disorganized. Lack of trained personnel, low salaries and incompetent officials, charged with crucial responsibilities for public health, seriously affected the efficiency of the entire organization. In addition, the Ministry of Welfare had not been permitted to assume its proper place in Japanese government and many of the activities generally associated with public health and welfare were the responsibilities of other Ministries. Upon the arrival of the Occupation Forces, Japanese public health and welfare activities were found to be in a very demoralized state. An

unsound administration, plus the nation's efforts to gear itself during the war, had completely broken down any semblance of health or welfare functions. (GHQ, SCAP, PHWS 1949a)

Assuming the relative accuracy of the SCAP evaluation, the rapid recovery and development of health and welfare administration and its subsequent contribution to the economic and health "miracles" is quite impressive. Although the Ministry of Health and Welfare (MHW) continues to share responsibility for health and welfare administration with other national and subnational agencies, it appears to have assumed the "proper place" in Japanese government that SCAP officials had in mind. It is an integral part of the extensive apparatus of state intervention in postwar Japanese society "for the promotion and extension of social welfare and security, and of public health" legitimated by Article 25.

In functional terms, Japanese national health administration may be divided into four main categories: (1) environmental protection, (2) industrial health administration, (3) school health administration, (4) general health administration. In each of these areas state intervention has led to the establishment of a complex administrative apparatus that is likely to grow in spite of the "administrative reform" policies adopted by recent prime ministers and cabinets. For example, state involvement in school health activities has increased in the postwar period. At the national level, the Ministry of Education, Science, and Culture is the state's main administrative agent and its Physical Education Bureau bears the major responsibility for preventive health programs in schools. Critics contend that state commitment to disease prevention and health promotion is weakest in the school health programs under the ministry's jurisdiction and that the school system must play a more important role in the future, not simply in promoting physical education and sports activities, but also in providing basic health education and fostering "good health habits" for school children (Sakuma 1978). Be that as it may, it should be noted that the high literacy rate and accumulated educational stock of the Japanese people as a result of the highly developed compulsory educational system has an important impact on the national state of health.

The story of the emergence of the Japanese version of the welfare state is fascinating but too complex to be told here.[6] It should be noted in passing, however, that the relevant activities of political parties and the organized interest groups of business, labor, providers, insurers, and the like, the roles of the legislative and judicial branches of Japanese government and, within the executive branch, the Economic Planning Agency and the Social Security System Council of the Office of the Prime Minister as well as the Ministry of Finance were all important components of the state in health, historically and at present. The discussion here will be limited to the current activities of the major national administrative agency concerned with health, the Ministry of Health and Welfare.

General health administration at the national level is centered in the Ministry of Health and Welfare. Established as a result of pressure from the military in 1938 and reorganized under the aegis of SCAP during the Occupation, the MHW was organized into nine bureaus, two departments, and one separate agency, and was responsible for 9.1 percent of the overall national budget in 1980. The ministry is engaged primarily in four types of activities: public health and medical care; social welfare and public aid; social insurance; and education, research, and information gathering. It oversees the administrative and programmatic activities of prefectural and city, town and village governments in the public health-medical care area as well as overseeing the system of health centers. The ministry also plays an important role in health planning and policy development at the national and regional levels. In general, the MHW is the most visible and concrete manifestation of the Japanese state in public health and medical care, and ministry officials are responsible for integration and coordination of health and medical affairs with other state activities and priorities.

The Medical Care Complex

As used here, "medical care" refers to the organization and delivery of personal health services, that is, diagnosis, treatment, rehabilitation, and prevention of disease and injury in individual cases. The providers and consumers of personal health services, the financing mechanisms, and the agencies through which state authority is exercised comprise the "medical care complex." Ostensibly, the bulk of personal health services are delivered through the private sector in contemporary Japan and financed through the system of comprehensive, compulsory health insurance. As previously indicated, however, the Japanese state is deeply involved in the organization and delivery of services, and the line between public and private sectors is not clearly drawn. State intervention in the medical care sector has a firm constitutional, historical, and cultural basis (Steslicke 1982b), and although countervailing forces are present, it seems likely that the role of the state will grow in coming years. A brief examination of the basic components of the medical care complex will indicate why.[7]

Medical Care Consumers

It has been argued that the state of physical, mental, and social well-being in contemporary Japan is among the highest in the world, in keeping with its status as the world's third major industrial power. However, economic development seems to generate as many health hazards as it eliminates. What is loosely referred to as "life-style" in the advanced industrial nations is sometimes seen as the key to health and illness, but is is not entirely clear whether this is a matter of individual choice or social determinants. There is also considerable disagreement as to whether the relatively affluent life-style in such nations is basically healthy or unhealthy or some combination of both. It is as easy in Japan as it is in the United States to stimulate a lively debate regarding life-style. What is clear in both countries, however, is that consumption of sophisticated, high-tech, professionalized medical services has become an intrinsic part of life for most of the population (Steslicke and Kimura 1985).

In 1981 more Japanese availed themselves of medical services than ever before. According to the annual patient survey conducted by the MHW, the rate increased from 4,805 per 100,000 persons receiving medical care on the survey date in 1960 to 7,049 per 100,000 in 1975. This proportion remained relatively stable between 1975 and 1980 (decreasing slightly to 6,855 per 100,000 in 1980), and peaked at 7,266 per 100,000 in 1981. The changing pattern in the illness categories for which care was sought between 1955 and 1981 is shown in the accompanying graph. Note especially the rise in hypertensive disease, heart diseases, and mental disorders. These trends are also likely to continue throughout the foreseeable future. Therefore, medical care providers can expect a healthy market for their services, particularly among the middle-aged and elderly segments of the population. Whether or not medical care providers have the personnel, skills, facilities, and credibility to adequately supply the changing needs and demands for medical services is problematic. This is generally recognized within the medical care community and, in order to cope with future circumstances, numerous public and private investigations are being conducted into various aspects of health care training and performance.

Medical Care Providers

Since the establishment of the system of medical care based on Western medical science following the Meiji Restoration, the provision of medical services has been restricted to individuals and organizations designated by the state. This state-supported monopoly has a statutory basis and is administered by government officials at the national and prefectural levels. Within the medical care monopoly, the physician has been authorized to dominate the division of labor. The various kinds of individual medical care providers and the requirements for entry into the exclusive circle are indicated in table 8. According to the Medical Practitioner's Law of July 30, 1948, as amended, only "duly licensed" individuals may use the title of "doctor" *(ishi)*, and are authorized to "take charge of medical treatment and guidance of health, and contribute to the improvement and promotion of public health in order to secure the healthy life of the people" (Art. 1). In 1980 there were 156,235 "duly

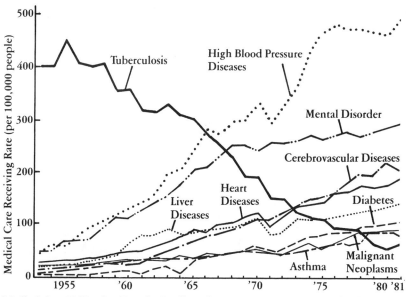

Medical Care Utilization Rate for Leading Illnesses per 100,000 Population in Japan, 1955–1981. From JICWELS (1983, 3).

Table 8. Types of Medical Care Providers and Licensure Requirements in Japan, 1980

	General Education			Professional Education		Examination	Licensed by
	Primary school (6 years)	Jr. high school (3 years)	Sr. high school (3 years)				
Medical doctor	XXXX	XXXX	XXXX	University Pre-med. (2 yrs.)	Professional (4 yrs.)	National	Minister for Health and Welfare
Dentist	XXXX	XXXX	XXXX	University Pre-dent. (2 yrs.)	" (4 yrs.)	" "	" "
Pharmacist	XXXX	XXXX	XXXX	University Pre-pharm. (2 yrs.)	" (2 yrs.)	" "	" "
Veterinarian	XXXX	XXXX	XXXX	University Pre-vet. (2 yrs.)	" (2 yrs.)	"	Minister of Agriculture and Forestry
Public health nurse (a)	XXXX	XXXX	XXXX	University (4 yrs.)		"	Minister for Health and Welfare
Public health nurse (b)	XXXX	XXXX	XXXX	Nursing school (3 yrs.)	PHN sch. (1 yr.)	"	"
Midwife (a)	XXXX	XXXX	XXXX	University (4 yrs.)		"	
Midwife (b)	XXXX	XXXX	XXXX	Nursing school (3 yrs.)	Midwife sch. (1 yr.)		
Clinical nurse (a)	XXXX	XXXX	XXXX	University (4 yrs.)		"	"
Clinical nurse (b)	XXXX	XXXX	XXXX	Nursing sch. (3 yrs.)		"	"
Clinical nurse (c)	XXXX	XXXX	Assistant nurse train. sch. (2 yrs.)	Practice (3 yrs.)	Nursing sch. (2 yrs.)	"	"

			Nursing high sch. course (3 yrs.)	Nursing School (2 yrs.)		Exam	Authority
Clinical nurse (d)	XXXX	XXXX	Nursing high sch. course (3 yrs.)	/		"	"
Assistant nurse (a)	XXXX	XXXX	Assistant nurse train. sch. (2 yrs.)			Prefectural Exam	Prefectural Governor
Assistant nurse (b)	XXXX	XXXX	Nursing high sch. course (3 yrs.)			"	"
Radiology technician	XXXX	XXXX	XXXX	School or training school (3 yrs.)	/	National	Minister for Health and Welfare
X-ray technician	XXXX	XXXX	XXXX	School or training school (2 yrs.)	/	"	"
Health laboratory technician	XXXX	XXXX	XXXX	(ditto)	/	"	"
Clinical laboratory technician	XXXX	XXXX	XXXX	School or training school (3 yrs.)	/	"	"
Physical therapist	XXXX	XXXX	XXXX	School or training school (3 yrs.)	/	"	"
Occupational therapist	XXXX	XXXX	XXXX	(ditto)	/	"	"
Dental hygienist	XXXX	XXXX	XXXX	School or training school (1–2 yrs.)	/	"	Prefectural Governor
Dental technician	XXXX	XXXX	XXXX	School or training school (2 yrs.)		Pref. Exam.	"
Nutritionist	XXXX	XXXX	XXXX	Training school (2, 3, 4 yrs.)	/	National	Minister for Health and Welfare

Source: Ministry of Health and Welfare (1981a, 20).

licensed" physicians, 53,502 dentists, and 487,169 nurses. (The distribution of these practitioners throughout the system is shown in table 9.)

In Japan, it is generally agreed that the most pressing personnel problem in the medical care sector is the acute shortage of nurses, including public health nurses. Of the latter, in 1980 the total number of 17,957 nurses represented 15.3 per 100,000 persons, that is, 6,519 persons for each public health nurse. There is no shortage in the total number of doctors, dentists, and pharmacists, but there is a very marked geographic maldistribution. There were 116,056 pharmacists in 1980, that is, 99.3 per 100,000 persons, or 1,009 persons per pharmacist (54.6 percent of pharmacists were females). The ratios of dentists and physicians were 45.8 and 133.6 per 100,000, respectively, or 2,184 persons per dentist

Table 9. Doctors, Dentists, and Nurses in Japan, 1960–1980

Practitioners	1960	1965	1970	1975	1980
Physicians					
Engaged in institutions:					
Employers in hospitals	2,449	2,608	3,597	3,250	3,468
Employers in clinics	47,849	52,609	57,170	59,904	61,646
Employees in hospitals	25,896	28,038	32,461	38,085	50,075
Employees in clinics	10,450	9,011	8,469	8,630	8,747
Employees in medical school hospitals	9,394	9,749	11,517	16,101	24,879
Engaged in non-institutions:					
Employees in medical schools	2,137	2,165	2,086	2,973	3,644
Administrative	2,632	2,260	1,895	2,067	2,099
Engaged in others	2,324	2,929	1,795	1,469	1,657
Total	103,131	109,369	118,990	132,479	156,235
Dentists	33,177	35,558	37,859	43,586	53,602
Nurses					
Engaged in nurses' schools	881	1,167	2,086	4,223	5,498
Engaged in health centers	325	317	357	430	493
Engaged in hospitals	144,575	189,021	213,880	279,316	377,746
Engaged in clinics	29,846	45,477	52,919	72,274	96,347
Engaged in schools	2,454	2,613	872	739	631
Dispatched nurses	6,370	5,488	974	948	518
Others	1,141	1,128	2,484	3,674	5,936
Total	185,592	245,211	273,572	361,604	487,169

Source: Ichijo and Kiikuni (1982, 13)

and 748 persons per physician. Of the physician population, 148,815, or 95.3 percent, were engaged in clinical practice and, of that number, 65,114, or 41.7 percent, were owners of hospitals and clinics. This means that, in 1980, 83,701 physicians in clinical practice, or 53.6 percent of the total, were salaried employees. A total of 24,879, or 15.9 percent of physicians, were employed in medical school hospitals. Thus, the majority of Japanese doctors are salaried employees working in hospitals, clinics, and other institutions, both public and private.

Despite their position as salaried employees, the practice of medicine remains highly regarded and well rewarded in contemporary Japan. There has been a rapid increase in medical school admissions in recent years, and it is estimated that the total number of physicians will increase by 50 percent in the next twenty years. By the year 2000 there would thus be 210 doctors and 81 dentists per 100,000 population. If the present pattern of geographical maldistribution persists, the already keen competition for customers will intensify. In recent years there have been a number of well-publicized scandals involving physicians and medical schools that have contributed to a growing sense of disenchantment with the medical establishment. Moreover, in their everyday relation with patients, many physicians have tended to reinforce the negative images popularized in the mass media. As a result, the medical mystique is losing a good deal of power and influence at both the individual and collective levels. Laypersons, both patients and public policymakers, no longer accept without question the notion that "doctor knows best." Clearly, the status and role of the physician in Japanese society is changing. Not only physicians, but all medical care providers are likely to encounter alterations in many phases of their work during the coming decades.

Medical Care Institutions

The dominant role of the physician in the provision of medical care is reinforced by the Medical Service Law of July 30, 1948, the basic governing statute for organization and delivery of medical services in Japan. The law distinguishes between "hospitals" and "clinics" by numbers of beds, the former having twenty or more beds and the latter nineteen or fewer. A "general hospital" is a facility of one hundred or more beds that also meets certain other specifications. According to the law, a hospital or clinic must be managed by a physician regardless of its ownership.

Table 10 gives the number of hospitals and clinics in Japan from 1965

Table 10. Number of Hospitals and Clinics in Japan, 1965–1980

Institutions	1965	1970	1975	1980
Hospitals				
General	5,922	6,869	7,235	8,003
Mental	725	896	929	977
Tuberculosis	340	160	87	39
Leprosy	14	14	16	16
Infectious	46	35	27	20
Total	7,047	7,974	8,294	9,005
Clinics				
With beds	27,332	29,841	29,104	28,956
Without beds	37,192	39,156	44,010	48,655
Total	64,524	68,997	73,114	77,611
Dental clinics	28,602	29,911	32,565	38,834

Source: Ichijo and Kiikuni (1982, 10).

Table 11. Number of Beds by Type of Hospital and Beds per 10,000 Population, 1965–1980

Beds	1965	1970	1975	1980
In hospitals				
General	442,536	601,978	721,858	895,494
Mental	172,950	247,265	278,123	308,554
Tuberculosis	220,757	176,949	129,055	84,905
Leprosy	13,230	13,217	14,020	12,235
Infectious	24,179	23,144	21,042	18,218
Total	873,652	1,062,553	1,164,098	1,319,406
Per 10,000 persons				
General	45.0	58.1	64.5	76.6
Mental	17.6	23.8	24.8	26.4
Tuberculosis	22.5	17.1	11.5	7.3
Leprosy	1.3	1.3	1.3	1.1
Infectious	2.5	2.2	1.9	1.6
Total	88.9	102.5	104.0	113.0

Source: Ichijo and Kiikuni (1982, 10).

to 1980. The number of beds in those hospitals and the beds per 10,000 persons over the same time span are shown in table 11 and the distribution of hospitals by type of ownership is indicated in table 12. It should be noted that when the 287,000 clinic beds are added to the 1,319,406 hospital beds in 1980, the bed-to-population ratio of 13.7 per 1,000 was 2.2 times as large as that of the United States.

For present purposes, but at the risk of considerable oversimplification, the following observations regarding medical care organization and delivery in contemporary Japan may be made. (1) Although there is a substantial "public sector" involvement in medical care, the bulk of medical services are delivered through the "private sector" (about 79 percent of the hospitals and 60 percent of the hospital beds and more than 90 percent of Japan's 77,000 clinics are privately owned and operated). (2) The delivery of services is highly competitive, with hospitals and clinics, both public and private, offering very similar services, resulting in considerable overlapping, redundancy, and excess capacity. (3) Since there are really no acute care hospitals as such and few special long-term care facilities, acute, chronic, short-term, long-term, inpatient, and outpatient care tends to be delivered in the same institutions for young and old alike, with a resulting average length of stay in hospitals of 38.3 days in 1980 as compared with 8 days in the United States (Goldsmith 1984, 119). (4) The closed-staff system means that every clinic and hospital is exclusive with respect to its patients and tries to offer "all-in-one" medical services. (5) Even though all Japanese physicians are specialists, most actually are engaged in general practice. (6) The quality of medical care is quite erratic, ranging from excellent to inferior, sometimes within

Table 12. Distribution of Hospitals in Japan by Type of Ownership, 1980

Ownership	Category of Hospitals					
	General	Mental	Tuber-culosis	Leprosy	Infectious disease	Total
National	437	3	0	13	0	453
Prefectural	259	37	6	0	1	303
Municipal	740	11	2	0	19	772
Other public	292	2	0	0	0	294
Social insurance	139	0	1	0	0	140
Private	6,136	924	30	3	0	7,093
Total	8,003	977	39	16	20	9,055

Source: Ichijo and Kiikuni (1982, 11).

the same facility. (7) The coordination and continuity of services from primary care to specialized care to rehabilitation and prevention are seriously deficient, and regional medical care planning is hampered by basic legal and structural constraints. (8) Since physicians are permitted both to dispense and prescribe drugs, overutilization of medicine has been a serious health hazard as well as a financial problem for consumers. (9) The trend toward high-technology medical care is well advanced, and the more or less traditional doctor-patient relationship has become severely strained as a consequence. (10) The combination of predominately private, fee-for-service, physician-centered medical care with compulsory, universal health insurance offering free choice of provider for insurees has created a serious financial crisis that currently seems to require substantial state intervention. This last component of the medical care complex merits more detailed examination.

Medical Care Financing

Perhaps the single most important feature of the medical care complex is the system of health insurance that has covered the entire population since 1961 (Steslicke 1982a). Based on the Health Insurance Law of 1922, the first of its kind in Asia, the system has grown incrementally to include other employment-based schemes for seamen, day laborers, teachers, and government workers. Citizens not covered by one of the employment-based schemes are entitled to coverage under the National Health Insurance Law of 1958, which requires that every city, town, or village in Japan offer health insurance to its residents and collect a special tax from those who are covered. Insurees are expected to share the costs of benefits with the community insurer and the national treasury.

The major features of the health insurance system are outlined in table 13. It is not necessary to go into the details of the various plans here except to note that there is a disparity in the level of benefits and cost sharing between the employment-based and community-based plans. Within the former category, members of society-managed plans tend to be much better off than members of government-managed schemes, many of which are chronically in the red. It is a complex system that reflects the politics of labor-management relations and the dual economy of modern Japan rather than the ideal of medical care planners for a more rational, efficient, and unified system. Efforts to reform the system in any fundamental way have been frustrated by the veto power exercised by the Japan Medical Association and other influential interest groups (Steslicke 1982b).

Table 13. Outline of Medical Care Insurance System in Japan, 1982

Scheme		Insured Persons	Insurer	Insurance Benefits				Financial Resources	
				Medical Care Benefits			Cash Benefits	Insurance Contribution	State Subsidy
				Medical Benefits	Dependents Medical Expenses	High-Cost Medical Care			
Health Insurance — Government-managed Health Insurance		Employees at places of work where health insurance societies are not established (small and medium size enterprises)	State	100% some cost-sharing	Inpatient 80% Outpatient 70%	Note: Patient cost-sharing ¥51,000. For low income persons, excess of ¥15,000	Injury and Sickness Allowance, Maternity Allowance, Childbirth Expenses	8.5% special benefits contribution—1% (Nov. 1981)	16.4% of benefit costs
Health Insurance — Society-managed Health Insurance		Employees at places of work where health insurance societies are established	Health Insurance Societies 1,703	100% (as above)	Inpatient 80% Outpatient 70% supplementary benefits exist	For low income persons, excess of ¥15,000	As above supplementary benefits exist	7.947% (average for all societies, 1980)	¥1,500 million as benefit cost assistance (1982)
Seamen's Insurance		Seamen (on designated vessels)	State	100% (as above)	Inpatient 80% Outpatient 70%	As above	As above	8.2% (Apr. 1982)	¥2,700 million as benefit cost assistance (1982)
Day Labourers' Health Insurance		Day Labourers { Employed on day-to-day basis, for fixed time less than 2 months, etc. }	State	100% (as above)	70%	Cost-sharing of ¥39,000	As above	Special Grade 1 —¥20 per day Grades 1–8 —¥60–¥660 per day	35% of benefit costs plus ¥600 million fixed sum (1982)
Mutual Aid Association Insurance — National Public Service MAAs		National public service employees	25 MAAs	100% (as above)	Inpatient 80% Outpatient 70%	As for Health Insurance	As above (supplementary benefits exist)	6.05–11.85% (Apr. 1981)	None
Mutual Aid Association Insurance — Local Public Service MAAs		Local public service employees	54 MAAs						
Mutual Aid Association Insurance — Public Corporation Employees MAAs		Employees of Japan National Railway, the Salt and Tobacco Monopoly, and Nippon Telephone and Telegraph	3 MAAs		Inpatient 80% Outpatient 70%				
Mutual Aid Association Insurance — Private School Teachers and Employees MAA		Private school teachers and employees	1 MAA						
Community Health Insurance — National Health Insurance		Those not covered by employees' insurance (agricultural workers, self-employed, construction workers, doctors, employees at small scale places of work)	Cities, Towns, Villages 3,272; National Health Insurance Associations 169	70% (both head of household and members) (benefit rate can be raised)		Cost-sharing ¥39,000; ¥39,000 for low income persons	Midwifery Expenses, Funeral Expenses, Nursing Allowance (optional)		45% of medical care costs plus temporary grant for financial adjustment 25–40% of medical care costs plus temporary adjustment assistance grant

Source: JICWELS (1983, 24).

From the standpoint of the individual citizen, the system offers relatively free access to medical services on an inpatient as well as on an outpatient basis without the fear that financial crisis will follow medical crisis. A much greater measure of medical security is available to the average Japanese citizen than to an American counterpart. From the standpoint of the provider, there is assurance not only that fees for service will be covered, but also that customers will be encouraged to enter the market for services quite freely. Providers are highly critical of many aspects of the system, even though they benefit from its operation. Mainly, they cry for increased payment under the unit-point system and for greater freedom within the national fee schedules that place many restrictions on treatment practices. Still, neither providers nor consumers are as disturbed as are insurers and payers at the rise in overall medical expenditures during the past decade.

In Japan, as in the United States and a number of other advanced industrial nations, cost containment has become the paramount concern in the medical care sector. Perhaps of somewhat less urgency in Japan than elsewhere, the situation is nevertheless serious. A summary of the basic facts is contained in table 14. By 1980 the rapid growth of medical care costs reached almost 12,000 billion yen, an estimated 4.98 percent of the GNP and 6.18 percent of national income. Because actual medical care expenditures may be underestimated by as much as 15 percent, according to some economists, it is of small comfort that the Japanese figures remain lower than in the United States and a number of other industrial nations. As indicated in a recent report from Japan: "During the period of high economic growth it was possible for the expanding economy to absorb the increase in medical care costs and they were not a matter for concern. However, following the oil shock, and even when the economy reverted to stable growth, medical care costs continued to rise at a faster pace than economic growth" (JICWELS 1983, 10). In short, it is not simply the rapid increase in medical costs but also the economic circumstances in which the increase has taken place that is troublesome.

How is the burden of medical costs distributed in contemporary Japan? In 1980 the national treasury's share was 30.5 percent, local government's share was 2.9 percent, and the insurance system's share was 54.5 percent, for a total of 88.2 percent. The remaining 11.8 percent was the direct patients' share of the burden. Whether or not a redistribution of shares is desirable or even possible is controversial. The question is

Table 14. Medical Care Costs in Japan, 1955-1980

Medical Care Costs

Year	Billion yen	Percentage increase over preceding year	Per-capita Costs yen	Medical Care Costs as Percentage		GNP billion yen	National Income billion yen
				of GNP	of NI		
1956	258.3	8.2	2,862	2.60	3.16	9,950.9	8,173.4
1958	323.0	11.5	3,511	2.74	3.36	11,785.0	9,616.1
1959	362.5	12.2	3,899	2.66	3.29	13,608.0	11,023.3
1960	409.5	13.0	4,384	2.53	3.09	16,207.0	13,269.1
1961	513.0	25.3	5,441	2.58	3.26	19,852.8	15,755.1
1962	613.2	19.5	6,443	2.83	3.46	21,659.5	17,729.8
1963	754.1	23.0	7,843	2.95	3.66	25,592.1	20,627.1
1964	938.9	24.5	9,661	3.17	4.01	29,661.9	23,390.4
1965	1,122.4	19.5	11,421	3.35	4.22	33,550.2	26,606.6
1966	1,300.2	15.8	13,126	3.30	4.18	39,452.0	31,106.6
1967	1,511.6	16.3	15,080	3.27	4.11	46,175.6	36,778.2
1968	1,801.6	19.2	17,766	3.29	4.18	54,689.2	43,126.0
1969	2,078.0	15.3	20,244	3.20	4.09	64,850.8	50,859.1
1970	2,496.2	20.1	24,032	3.32	4.10	75,091.6	60,875.4
1971	2,725.0	9.2	25,949	3.29	4.14	82,725.8	65,845.6
1972	3,399.4	24.7	31,672	3.53	4.38	96,424.0	77,602.1
1973	3,949.6	16.2	36,332	3.39	4.13	116,636.3	95,526.0
1974	5,378.6	36.2	48,875	3.90	4.80	138,044.6	112,081.6
1975	6,477.9	20.4	57,781	4.27	5.26	151,797.0	123,184.3
1976	7,668.4	18.4	67,810	4.50	5.54	172,900.1	138,446.8
1977	8,568.6	11.7	75,100	4.54	5.61	188,804.3	152,690.2
1978	10,004.2	16.8	86,900	4.84	6.00	206,762.5	166,854.9
1979	10,951.0	9.5	94,300	4.93	6.13	222,043.1	178,712.5
1980	11,980.5	9.4	102,300	4.98	6.18	240,647.0	193,811.7
1981	12,870.9	7.4	109,200	5.07	6.36	253,811.2	202,429.6

Source: Ichijo and Kiikuni (1982, 18)

highly political and is being debated in that arena. A partial answer has been incorporated into the recently passed Health and Medical Care Services for the Elderly Law (Rōjin Hoken-Hō). Increasing the patient's share may be the trend of the future, but resistance may prove quite fierce. Under the circumstances, providers can expect increasing pressure to join the battle, largely at their own expense. Thus, rationalization of medical care costs is likely to produce among various components of the medical care complex a struggle that will force a change in the strategy of state intervention developed during the happier days of high economic growth. Government officials at the national level are eagerly preparing themselves to serve as the agents of a new strategy of state intervention.

Medical Care and Government

As stated earlier, the Japanese state has been involved in health care since the early 1870s, and government has been a basic component of the medical care complex at both national and regional levels. The specific form, content, and magnitude of government involvement have, of course, changed over time (Steslicke 1972). Since its establishment in 1938, the Ministry of Health and Welfare has been the major national government agency responsible for medical care policy and administration.

Within the MHW, four bureaus are most closely concerned with medical care policy and administration. They are the Health Policy Bureau, the Pharmaceutical Affairs Bureau, the Health Service Bureau, and the Health Insurance Bureau. Many of the career officials assigned to the four bureaus are graduates of medical and other health-related schools and bring some measure of scientific or technical expertise to their bureaucratic positions, though the majority of MHW officials have followed the more conventional path to career service and are graduates of the law departments of Tokyo University or other national universities. Although difficult to document, it is clear that ideological and programmatic differences do exist within the MHW and that officials have competing interests and loyalties, as well as differing postretirement aspirations. There is also a surprising degree of fragmentation and lack of coordination between bureaus. Still, in a basic structural sense, MHW officials share a common interest in promoting the role of the ministry in the overall governmental process and in enhancing their own stature as managers of state intervention in the medical care system. They may not be in a very good position to set basic priorities for the nation, but they do seek to articulate those priorities within the medical care complex.

The Health Care Industry

The medical care complex is expected to contribute to the general well-being of the Japanese population while at the same time providing psychic and material rewards to service providers. However, the medical care complex is also part of a much larger and expanding health care industry. While the medical care complex is legally organized on a not-for-profit basis, other components of the health care industry are expected to provide a return to investors and to contribute to general economic health and well-being. This is especially true of producers of pharmaceutical and medical/dental instruments and supplies. In Japan, as in other advanced capitalist societies, the production and distribution of goods and services related to health has become big business, not only for domestic consumption, but also for foreign export. A brief examination of these two subsectors of the health care industry is illustrative.

In 1980 the total value of finished pharmaceutical products was estimated at 3,482,177 million yen, a new high that was a 14.5 percent increase over 1979 production. Since 1979 production had increased by only 8.9 percent over 1978, the return to double-digit growth was welcomed within the industry, even though it was far less than the record growth of 20.6 percent of 1976 (13.7 percent for 1977 and 1978). As in 1979, the major products were antibiotics (23.4 percent of the total) followed by cardiovascular products (see table 15). Although total growth in 1980 was mainly attributed to the rapid growth of the major pharmacotherapeutic categories listed in table 15, it is interesting to note that production of Chinese medicines also increased by 23 percent, even though their market share was a mere 1 percent of the total.

The overwhelming dominance in the production and sale of prescription drugs over nonprescription drugs was secured by a 16.3 percent increase in production in 1980. Nonprescription drugs increased in output by 4.9 percent, but their market share fell from 15.8 percent in 1979 to 14.5 percent in 1980. The share of prescription drugs in the total drug market was 85.5 percent in 1980. As indicated in table 16, sales of the sixteen major pharmaceutical companies totaled 1,684,183 million yen for fiscal years ending in 1980 or 1981, a 10 percent increase over the 1979–1980 period. Profits of 77,282 million yen were higher by 8 percent in spite of the 19,900 million yen paid by Takeda and Tanabe Seiyaku as compensation to victims of SMON (subacute myelo-opthalmoneuropathy, an iatrogenic disease resulting from a drug prescribed for various gastrointestinal problems. Subsidiaries and Japanese affiliates of foreign drug companies also did well in 1980. Those with sales of 30 billion yen or more included Ciba-Geigy (Japan) Ltd., the Sandoz group, Hoechst Japan Ltd., and No. 1 Pfizer Taito Company.

In more recent times, several major facts stand out. First, until the early 1960s, the industry concentrated on domestic production and sales of products that had been developed abroad; by 1980, it was estimated that about 40 percent of the drugs produced domestically were developed by the Japanese. Also, in 1980, drug exports reached a high of 93,901 million yen, an increase of 12.5 percent over 1979. Although this

Table 15. Pharmaceutical Production by Pharmacotherapeutic Category in 1979 and 1980

Rank in 1980	Category	Total Production 1979 (¥1 mil)	Total Production 1980 (¥1 mil)	1980 Change from 1979 Value (¥1 mil)	1980 Change from 1979 Rate (%)	Ratio to Total 1979 (%)	Ratio to Total 1980 (%)
1	Antibiotics	658,009	814,320	156,311	23.8	21.6	23.4
2	Cardiovasculars	309,332	377,757	68,425	22.1	10.2	10.8
3	Miscellaneous agents affecting metabolism	315,601	363,950	48,349	15.3	10.4	10.5
4	Agents affecting central nervous system	304,503	344,197	39,694	13.0	10.0	9.9
5	Agents affecting digestive organs	240,960	256,830	15,870	6.6	7.9	7.4
6	Vitamins	210,813	216,249	5,436	2.6	6.9	6.2
7	Agents for epidermis	189,942	197,984	8,042	4.2	6.2	5.7
8	Biologicals	91,533	114,396	22,863	25.0	3.0	3.3
9	Antineoplastics	93,782	107,351	13,569	14.5	3.1	3.1
10	Hormones	82,986	89,315	6,329	7.6	2.7	2.6
11	Nutrients, tonics, and alternatives	82,684	85,704	3,020	3.7	2.7	2.5
12	Agents relating to blood and body fluids	71,577	82,690	11,113	15.5	2.4	2.4
13	Agents affecting peripheral nervous system	81,944	80,272	-1,672	-2.0	2.7	2.3
14	Agents affecting respiratory organs	67,257	79,960	12,703	18.9	2.2	2.3
15	Agents affecting sensory organs	41,070	45,005	3,929	9.6	1.4	1.3
16	Antiallergics	30,744	35,985	5,241	17.0	1.0	1.0
17	Agents for urogenital and anal organs	28,567	34,573	6,006	21.0	0.9	1.0
18	Chinese medicines	27,432	33,749	6,317	23.0	0.9	1.0
19	Diagnostics	28,059	30,164	2,105	7.5	0.9	0.9
20	Chemotherapeutics	29,940	29,487	-453	-1.5	1.0	0.8
21	Agents for public health	20,126	19,918	-208	-1.0	0.7	0.6
22	Agents for dispensing use	13,849	14,995	1,146	8.3	0.5	0.4
23	Agents for treatment and diagnosis of tissue cells	8,481	12,390	3,909	46.1	0.3	0.4
24	Agents for artificial dialysis	6,097	7,137	1,040	17.1	0.2	0.2
25	Agents against parasites	1,866	1,884	18	1.0	0.1	0.1
26	Agents activating cellular function	2,068	1,750	-318	-15.4	0.1	0.1
	All others	3,076	4,165	1,089	35.4	0.1	0.1
	Total	3,042,302	3,482,177	439,875	14.5	100.0	100.0

Source: Japan Medical Gazette (Dec. 20, 1981, 4).

Table 16. Sales and Net Profits of 16 Major Pharmaceutical Companies in Japan, 1979 and 1980

Company	Sales				Net Profits			
	Fiscal year ended in '79 or '80		Fiscal year ended in '80 or '81		Fiscal year ended in '79 or '80		Fiscal year ended in '80 or '81	
	Value (¥1 mil)	Annual change (%)	Value (¥1 mil)	Annual change (%)	Value (¥1 mil)	Annual change (%)	Value (¥1 mil)	Annual change (%)
Takeda (1871)	420,316	13	430,883	3	16,428	20	17,447[a]	6
Sankyo (1899)	159,925	22	187,196	17	5,432	73	6,841	26
Fujisawa (1894)	139,206	10	155,906	12	13,492	12	13,862	3
Shionagi	132,692	11	142,304	7	7,969	1	8,039	1
Tanabe Seiyaku (1678)	106,111	8	114,544	8	-3,902	-893	-4,245[b]	-9
Eisai (1941)	92,024	11	103,365	12	5,627	24	6,115	9
Yamanouchi	68,568	11	76,601	12	4,689	43	5,556	18
Daiichi Seiyaku (1915)	66,625	11	73,596	10	3,289	19	3,514	7
Chugai (1943)	65,136	13	71,353	10	3,535	18	4,160	18
Banyu (1915)	55,873	10	64,116	15	2,700	2	2,709	0.3
Dainippon (1897)	47,812	10	53,195	11	1,123	-13	1,265	13
Yoshitomi	41,208	-4	44,106	7	1,287	-0.2	1,001	-0.2
Green Cross (1950)	45,544	24	59,962	32	3,900	34	4,528	16
Mochida	35,705	18	40,559	14	3,600	27	3,889	8
Nippon Shinyaku (1919)	32,685	11	34,636	6	1,479	10	1,648	11
Toyama (1936)	28,032	-2	31,865	14	755	-17	912	21
Total and Average	1,537,392	12	1,684,183	10	71,402	13	77,282	8

Source: Japan Medical Gazette (Nov. 20, 1981, 1).

[a] Reserve of ¥3,500 million for SMON dispute.

[b] Compensation of ¥12,402 million and reserve of ¥4,000 million for SMON dispute.

figure was only about 2.5 percent of total production and a mere 0.3 percent of total Japanese exports, the internationalization process is well underway, and Japan has become part of the "multinationalization" of the pharmaceutical industry. Imports were also up by 19.9 percent in 1980 (0.8 percent of total Japanese imports) and exceeded exports by over 168,000 million yen. A second important fact for the industry is that the health insurance system that stimulated growth and development in the 1960s and 1970s is now forcing substantial reorganization of the way the pharmaceutical industry does business in Japan. A downward revision of an average of 18.6 percent in the health insurance standard prices by the Ministry of Health and Welfare in 1981—with more downward revisions in the offing—was one of those "shocks" that seem to hit so often in Japan. A third fact affecting the industry is the emergence of biotechnology and corresponding new frontiers for exploration and international competition during the 1980s. Much is expected of the industry in this arena by investors, medical care providers, consumers, and the agents of the Japanese developmental state (Kasagi 1982, 112).

Although of much more recent vintage as a recognized subsector of the health care industry, ME (a designation often used in Japan) is also seen as an attractive investment opportunity for the 1980s. ME is used in three different ways at present (Konagaya 1982, 100). The narrowest usage means "medical electronics," including electronic machinery, apparatus, and equipment such as X ray, CT (computer tomographic) devices, ultrasonic diagnostic devices, automatic biochemical analysis equipment, urinal dialysis devices, and nuclear diagnostic devices. ME is also used more broadly to mean "medical engineering," thereby including a wider range of medical and dental instruments and supplies. The third and broadest definition of ME used by the MHW in its annual statistical reports embraces the full range of medical equipment as categorized in table 17. As indicated, 1980 production totaled 720,184 million yen, an all-time high and an increase of 27 percent over 1979 production. It is not surprising that "devices for hospitals and clinics" tops the list and represents 25.7 percent of the total. "Diagnostic instruments and apparatus" (11.6 percent) and "related goods for radioactivity" (11.6 percent) are second and third, with the latter showing a spectacular increase of 85.1 percent over 1979. The bulk of production in that category is of X ray photographic film. ME production and sales figures demonstrate that high technology medicine has arrived in Japan.

This development is even more striking when viewed in terms of the

Table 17. Production of Medical Equipment in Japan, 1979 and 1980

Category	1979 Value (¥1 mil)	1979 % to total	1980 Value (¥1 mil)	1980 % to total	% change from '79
Devices for hospitals and clinics	151,729	26.8	185,044	25.7	22.0
Steel products for medical use	4,009	0.7	4,634	0.6	15.6
Diagnostic instruments and apparatus	64,259	11.3	83,802	11.6	30.4
Operating instruments and apparatus	28,077	5.0	39,131	5.4	39.4
Devices for medical treatment	38,692	6.8	60,623	8.4	56.7
Laboratory instruments and apparatus	2,629	0.5	2,474	0.3	-5.9
Instruments and apparatus for dental consulting room	28,729	5.1	32,034	4.4	11.5
Instruments and apparatus for dental consulting	5,685	1.0	6,421	0.9	12.9
Related goods for radioactivity	44,884	7.9	83,069	11.5	85.1
Sutures	2,087	0.4	2,392	0.3	14.6
Surgical goods, orthopedic goods, and related products	12,842	2.3	13,589	1.9	5.8
Ophtholmic goods	44,548	7.9	48,899	6.8	9.8
Hearing aids	4,491	0.8	5,280	0.7	17.6
Simplified therapeutic instruments	57,590	10.2	70,237	9.8	22.0
Dental materials	63,983	11.3	68,810	9.6	7.5
Birth control products	7,277	1.3	7,908	1.1	8.7
Others	5,412	1.0	5,838	0.8	7.9
Total	566,922	100.0	720,184	100.0	27.0

Source: Japan Medical Gazette (Dec. 20, 1981, 2).

narrow definition of ME (medical electronics) used in Ministry of International Trade and Industry (MITI) statistics, which report total ME production for 1980 to be roughly 250,000 million yen, a 20 percent plus increase over 1979. This branch of the industry, which is less than twenty years old, consists of about twenty fiercely competitive Japanese firms, mainly large electric and electronic manufacturers such as Hitachi and Toshiba that produce ME as a sideline, plus a few foreign participants in the field.

The 1980s were also a kind of crossroads for this branch of the ME industry. After ten years of boom, the medical care complex has become saturated with its products. This circumstance has intensified competition and has led to the underpricing of many products, thus encouraging grossly inappropriate utilization. During the latter half of 1980, a series of exposés of overuse, misuse, and abuse of ME products in various hospitals and clinics caused grave concern even among medical care providers themselves. Also, the 18.6 percent decrease in the standard price of drugs of June 1981 and other MHW efforts at rationalization of medical care costs have had a sobering effect on medical care providers who had gotten into the habit of reinvesting income derived from drugs and ME back into new ME equipment. Nevertheless, the ME boom is unlikely to collapse in the foreseeable future, and internationalization of the industry will probably continue at a rapid pace.

Health and Medical Care Policy in the 1980s

The Japanese developmental state played a major role in promoting economic recovery and growth in the postwar era, thereby contributing to the generally high levels of health and well-being of the population at the beginning of the 1980s. Direct state intervention in public health and medical care has also contributed to economic recovery and growth, and government has become a basic component of the contemporary medical care complex. What government does or does not do has an important bearing on the organization, financing, and delivery of medical care as well as on the general state of health. Although national policymakers are preoccupied with various pressing issues related to defense, trade, and the changing domestic and international economies, it has become impossible for them to ignore the signs and symptoms of distress in the medical care sector. Articulation of the health policy agenda for the future has become an urgent but controversial matter.

The controversy has intensified the ongoing struggle for power and prestige in the medical care complex between various interested groups and individuals. There are about forty national associations representing providers, insurers, business, and labor that are active in the medical care policy arena. Although none of these associations directly and unequivocally represent medical care consumers as such, most claim to represent the public interest.

Officials of the major associations interact both formally and informally with each other as well as with elected and appointed government and political party officials. It is a relatively stable network of full-time professionals who see each other in Diet committee meetings, advisory council sessions, public and private study groups, task forces, seminars and social gatherings, and other institutionalized channels for communication and decision making. Informally the network has a decided "old boy" character. Moreover, in keeping with Japanese tradition, the *amakudari* (descent from heaven) practice is followed, whereby top bureaucrats are moved into lucrative retirement jobs, and current MHW officials, for example, find themselves dealing with former associates and superiors who have become Dietmen or group officials. It is a network in which there are few strangers and in which the battle lines are well known and respected. As in other policy arenas, a number of active and retired academicians have become regulars who sometimes exercise considerable influence; however, their main role is to provide expert information and advice and help to legitimize the innumerable "deals" of which medical care policy has been composed.

This more or less "normal" policy-making process emerged from the bitter struggles of the late 1950s and early 1960s, when the Japan Medical Association, led by Dr. Takemi Taro, strongly contested implementation of the government's universal health insurance program (Steslicke 1973). Negotiations involving high-level cabinet and Liberal Democratic party officials and the various contending interest groups led to a compromise agreement that averted the threatened general resignation from health insurance practice by JMA members. For the next two decades MHW officials, in cooperation with key Liberal Democratic party Dietmen and staff, assumed responsibility for maintaining the uneasy truce by accommodating and balancing the interests and demands of the various contending forces. While their broad objective was to promote the national priorities articulated in the series of economic and social plans and other basic policy pronouncements (mainly economic productivity and social stability), the more immediate objective was to manage the conflicts and contradictions within the medical care complex.

The most troublesome aspect of this for state managers has been the health insurance system. In order to keep the system working for providers, insurers, and consumers of medical care, it was necessary to arrange a series of compromises. When the deals were made, whether formally or informally, representatives of the leading national associations participated in the process of negotiations, consultations, conferences, and bargaining sessions that became quite routinized and ritualized. The process closely resembled the "limited pluralism" characterizing many other public-policy arenas in Japan during the 1960s and 1970s (Fukui 1972, 1977).

By the late 1970s it became clear that the broader economic and social context of health and medical care was changing (Economic Planning Agency 1979, 1). Under the circumstances, the problems within the medical care complex that were so well managed and contained during the preceding era of recovery and high growth became more troublesome. In order to cope with the realities of the new era, policymakers have been forced to abandon the essentially passive and accommodationist approach to state intervention and to adopt a more active, developmental strategy. Given the persistence of the limited-pluralism pattern in the medical care policy arena, wherein even marginal, incremental reforms are not easily induced, more basic structural changes should prove extremely difficult; yet, such changes may be necessary. Policymakers will also be forced to contend with the growing sense of entitlement to accessible, high quality, and affordable medical care within the populace, especially among the elderly.

This bottom-up expression of concern for health is shared by national policymakers. The emphasis at the top, however, is not so much on personal health as on fiscal health. Fiscal reconstruction and administrative reform are top priorities on the domestic policy agenda, and the national health insurance system has been targeted as a major source of budgetary distress requiring remedial action. These priorities are strongly supported within the corporate establishment. Demands by leading business associations for reform of the nation's health insurance system, so as to contain costs and discourage overutilization of medical services, will increase the sense of urgency within the government. Management also is demanding increased cost sharing by workers for their own and their dependents' health insurance and medical care (Steslicke 1984).

The Japan Medical Association has advocated a more fundamental reorganization of the health insurance system in the direction of a single, unified, community-based system along the lines of the National Health Insurance Law. The JMA has maintained its strong support for private practice, fee-for-service medical care and has resisted all government efforts to experiment with capitation reimbursement methods. Under Dr. Takemi's leadership, the JMA called for "denationalization" of health insurance and the institution of a privately managed system of "bio-insurance." Dr. Takemi retired as JMA president in 1982 and died in 1983.[8] It is not clear to what extent the current JMA leadership will actively support its inherited positions or develop a more compliant stance vis-à-vis the ongoing reform efforts directed by MHW officials.

Perhaps the major accomplishment of the reform effort thus far was the enactment of the Health Care for the Aged Law in August of 1982. Skeptics have dismissed as more symbolic than tangible the changes the new legislation introduced in the system of health and medical care for Japan's rapidly aging population (Campbell 1984, 1979). Supporters of the law prefer to see it as the "first step" in the direction of a more comprehensive reorganization and reorientation of health and medical services in Japan that will emphasize disease prevention and health promotion as well as high-technology, cure-oriented medical intervention (JICWELS 1983, 18). Implementation of the complex new system provided for in the law is, therefore, one of the top priorities on the MHW agenda. The long-term rationalization of medical costs is contingent upon some degree of success in that effort.

What the state does or does not do in the health and medical care arena and how the public policy agenda is formulated and implemented in the coming years is of enormous interest and concern in Japan. However, it should also be of considerable interest in the United States and other industrial nations. After all, the state of health is not a purely domestic concern within particular nations—especially for those who must compete in the international marketplace for goods and services in order to survive. A nation's state of health and the way in which health and medical care services are organized and delivered has a significant bearing on productive capacity and costs. Japanese leaders would very much like to maintain the relative advantage the nation has had in that respect during the past few decades by dealing with current medical care problems before they get out of control. Although they are placing emphasis on "the vitality of the private sector" *(minkan katsuryoku)* as a way of coping with such problems, they will continue to rely on state intervention in the health care system as in the past.

Notes

1. Consider, for example, the following description as a frame of reference.

At the time of Japan's surrender in August 1945, the nation was confronted with the awesome costs of the war. Combined military and civilian casualties totalled about 1,800,000 dead; civilians alone accounted for 668,000 killed, wounded or missing; roughly twenty-five percent of the national wealth had been destroyed or lost; some forty percent of the built-up area of the sixty-six major cities subjected to air attacks had been leveled to the ground; about twenty percent of the nation's residential housing and almost twenty-five percent of all her buildings were obliterated; thirty percent of her industrial capacity, eighty percent of her shipping, and forty-seven percent of her thermal power-generating capacity were destroyed; forty-six percent of her prewar territory had been lost, some of it only temporarily, however. Other more intangible costs were harder to calculate: the long-term economic significance of the loss of Empire; the political consequences of being reduced to the status of a second-or-third-class power; the effects of being cut off from established trading partners; the consequences of facing world suspicion and opposition to any revival of Japan's prewar eminence in Eastern Asia. Japan's immediate prospects were ominous and alarming. What had become of the country? How was it to be reconstructed and rehabilitated? (Ward 1967, 17–18)

Ohtani (1971, 7–107) gives a brief description of the state of health and the health care system in the immediate postwar period. For a more detailed account of that period, see GHQ, SCAP, PHWS 1949a, 1949b.

2. Chalmers Johnson (1982, 305–306) writes:

The effectiveness of the Japanese state in the economic realm is to be explained in the first instance by its priorities. For more than 50 years the Japanese state has given its first priority to economic development. This does not mean that the state has always been effective in achieving its priorities throughout this period, but the consistency and continuity of its top priority generated a learning process that made the state much more effective during the second half of the period than the first. . . . A state attempting to match the economic achievements of Japan must adopt the same priorities as Japan. It must first of all be a developmental state—and only then a regulatory state, a welfare state, an equality state, or whatever other kind of functional state a society may wish to adopt. This commitment to development does not, of course, guarantee any particular degree of success; it is merely prerequisite.

3. By "state of health" I mean to suggest somatic, psychic, and social aspects of national "health" (well-being) in a broad international and historical perspective. However, the actual description is a crude and eclectic review of mortality and morbidity data that is not intended to be definitive. It is more or less in keeping with the following observation. As defined in the constitution of the World Health Organization:

"health is a state of complete physical, mental and social well-being and not merely the absence of disease or infirmity." Unfortunately, health status cannot be adequately measured in such terms anywhere in the world. It is still common, indeed necessary, to measure and compare health primarily in terms of the incidence and prevalence of diseases or infirmities, variations in causes of death, and according to levels and trends in mortality. For the most part the available data on health status for the less developed countries range from the extremely weak to the non-existent. Information on morbidity and cause of death is often only accurate within very broad ranges of error for the more developed countries. Similarly, both time-series data and statistics from different countries are frequently not fully comparable. Consequently, health status differentials can only be discussed in broad terms. (WHO 1980, 37)

See also Goldsmith (1972, 212–221) and Jazairi (1976). For a Japanese approach, see Research Committee, Council of National Living (1975, 87–136).

4. According to the WHO report:

Life expectancy at birth, despite its limitations, has time and again been proved to be the most important single measure of the level of health of a population, particularly when viewed from the broader perspective of socioeconomic development strategy. A study made by the United Nations Research Institute for Social Development has found that life expectancy was closely correlated with the "general development index" devised by the Institute, and much more substantially so than any other available health status indicators. Even in developed countries the correlation between gross national product per capita, used as a proxy indicator of economic development, and life expectancy at birth is still highly significant. (WHO 1980, 238)

5. A more complete description would include what Henrik L. Blum (1981, 15–16) proposes as "twelve measurable aspects of the state of health," that is, (1) life span, (2) disease or infirmity, (3) discomfort or illness, (4) disability or incapacity, (5) participation in health care, (6) health behavior, (7) ecologic behavior, (8) social behavior, (9) interpersonal relationships, (10) reserve or positive health, (11) external satisfaction, and (12) internal satisfaction.

6. Some useful accounts of the development of the health and medical care components of the Japanese welfare state include: Kōseishō 1953, 1955, 1960, 1980; Nakano 1976; Ohtani 1971; Kawakami 1977; Saguchi 1960, 1985; Lock 1980; and Steslicke (1972).

7. Among the many annual publications in Japanese that offer statistical and other descriptive information and documents related to health and medical care, the following are especially convenient and useful: Kenkō Hoken Kumiai Rengōkai (1982), Kōsei Tōkei Kyōkai (1983a, 1983b, 1985), and Kōseishō (1983).

8. Dr. Takemi was quite prolific and a collection of some of his writings is now available in English (see Takemi 1982).

References

Abel-Smith, B. 1976. *Value for money in health services.* London: William Heinemann.

Bennett, J. W., and S. B. Levine. 1976. Industrialization and social deprivation. In *Japanese industrialization and its social consequences,* ed. H. Patrick. Berkeley and Los Angeles: Univ. of California Press.

Blum, H. L. 1981. *Planning for health.* New York: Human Science Press.

Campbell, J. C. 1979. The old people boom and Japanese policy making. *Journal of Japanese Studies* 5:321–357.

———. 1984. Problems, solutions, and non-solutions, and free medical care for the elderly in Japan. *Pacific Affairs* 57:53–64.

Caudill, W. 1976. The cultural and interpersonal context of everyday health and illness in Japan and America. In *Asian medical systems,* ed. C. Leslie. Berkeley and Los Angeles: Univ. of California Press.

Economic Planning Agency, Govt. of Japan. 1979. *New economic and social seven-year plan.* Tokyo: Ministry of Finance.

———. 1981. *In search of a good quality of life.* Tokyo: Ministry of Finance.

Environment Agency, Govt. of Japan. 1982. *Quality of the environment in Japan 1981.* Tokyo: Health Welfare and Environment Problems Research Society.

Fukui, H. 1972. Economic planning in postwar Japan. *Asian Survey* 12:327–348.

———. 1977. Studies in policymaking. In *Policymaking in contemporary Japan,* ed. T. J. Pempel. Ithaca: Cornell Univ. Press.

General Headquarters, Supreme Commander for the Allied Powers, Public Health and Welfare Section (GHQ, SCAP, PHWS). 1949a. *Public health and welfare in Japan.*

———. 1949b. *Public health and welfare in Japan, annex and charts.*

Goldsmith, S. B. 1972. The status of health care indicators. *Health Services—Reports* 82:212–221.

———. 1984. *Theory Z hospital management.* Rockville, Md.: Aspen Systems Corporation.

Hashimoto, M. 1981. National health administration in Japan. *Bulletin of the Institute for Public Health* 30:1–26.

Huddle, N., and M. Reich. 1975. *Island of dreams.* New York and Tokyo: Autumn Press.

Ichijo, K., and K. Kiikuni. 1982. Health services in Japan. *Japan-Hospitals: The Journal of the Japan Hospital Association* 1:3–30.

Iga, M., et al. 1978. Suicide in Japan. Special issue, Social science and medicine in Japan. *Social Science and Medicine* 12:507–516.

Ikegami, N. 1982. The institutionalized and the non-institutionalized elderly. *Social Science and Medicine* 16:2001–2008.

Institute of Administrative Management, Administrative Management Agency, Prime Minister's Office, Govt. of Japan. 1981. *Organization of the government of Japan.* Tokyo: IAM.

Japan Institute of Labor. 1982. *Japanese industrial relations series: Industrial safety and health.* Tokyo: JIL.

Japan International Corporation of Welfare Services (JICWELS). 1983. *Trends and policies of health care services in Japan.* Tokyo: JICWELS.

Japan Medical Gazette. Nov. 20 and Dec. 20, 1981.

Jazairi, N. T. 1976. *Approaches to the development of health indicators*. Paris: OECD.

Johnson, C. 1982. *MITI and the Japanese miracle*. Stanford: Stanford Univ. Press.

Kasagi, M. 1982. Pharmaceutical industry faces two difficulties. In *Industrial Review of Japan/1982*, ed. *Japan Economic Journal*. Tokyo: Nihon Keizai Shimbun.

Kawakami, T. 1977. *Gendai Nihon iryōshi* (The history of modern Japanese medicine). 8th ed. Tokyo: Chikuma Shobo.

Kenkō Hoken Kumiai Rengōkai. 1982. *Shakai hoshō nenkan 1982* (Social security yearbook 1982). Tokyo.

Konagaya, T. 1982. Medical equipment. In *Industrial review of Japan/1982*, ed. *Japan Economic Journal*. Tokyo: Nihon Keizai Shimbun.

Kōseishō. 1983. *Kōsei hakusho* (Health and welfare white paper). Tokyo: Okurasho Insatsukyoku.

Kōseishō Hokenkyoku, ed. 1953. *Kenkō hoken nijūgonen-shi* (Twenty-five year history of health insurance). Tokyo: Zenkoku Shakai Hokenkyoku Rengōkai.

———. 1980. *Kokumin kenkō hoken yonjūnen-shi* (Forty-year history of national health insurance.) Tokyo: Kabushikigaisha Gyosei.

Kōseishō Imukyoku, ed. 1955. *Isei hachijūnen-shi* (Eighty-year history of medical administration). Tokyo: Okurashu Insatsukyokyu.

Kōseishō Nijūnen-shi Henshu Iinkai, ed. 1960. *Kōseishō nijūnen-shi* (Twenty-year history of the Ministry of Health and Welfare). Tokyo: Kōsei Mondai Kenkyukai.

Kōsei Tōkei Kyōkai. 1983a. *Hoken to nenkin no dōkō* (Trends in health insurance and pensions). Tokyo.

———. 1983b. *Kokumin eisei no dōkō* (Trends in national public health). Tokyo.

———. 1985. *Kokumin no fukushi no dōkō* (Trends in national welfare). Tokyo.

Kubota, J. 1980. Occupational health in Japan. *Asian Medical Journal* 23:308–318.

Lock, M. M. 1980. *East Asian medicine in urban Japan*. Berkeley and Los Angeles: Univ. of California Press.

Ministry of Health and Welfare. 1981a. Guide to health and welfare services in Japan. Tokyo: Health and Welfare Problems Research Society.

———. 1981b. Outline of the 1980 national health survey. Tokyo: Foreign Press Center.

Nakano, H. 1976. *Gendai Nihon no ishi* (Modern Japanese physicians). Tokyo: Nikkei Shinsho.

National Federation of Health Insurance Societies (KEMPOREN). 1984. *Health insurance and health insurance societies in Japan*. Tokyo: KEMPOREN.

Ogawa, N. 1982. Economic implications of Japan's aging population. *International Labor Review* 12:117–133.

Ohtani, F. 1971. *One hundred years of health progress in Japan*. Tokyo: International Medical Foundation of Japan.

Public Health Bureau, Ministry of Health and Welfare. 1980. Future cancer prevention measures in Japan. Report of the cancer prevention measures discussion committee, July 1980.

Reich, M. R. 1983a. Environmental policy and Japanese society, part 1. *International Journal of Environmental Studies* 20:191–198.

———. 1983b. Environmental policy and Japanese society, part 2. *International Journal of Environmental Studies* 20:199–207.

Reich, M. R., and J. J. Kao. 1979. *A comparative view of health and medicine in Japan and America*. New York: Japan Society.

Renaud, M. 1975. On the structural constraints to state intervention in health. *International Journal of Health Services* 5:559–571.

Research Committee, Council of National Living. 1975. *Social indicators of Japan*. Tokyo: Ministry of Finance.

Saguchi, T. 1960. *Nihon shakai hoken-shi* (History of social insurance in Japan). Tokyo: Nihon Hyoron Shinsha.

———. 1985. Nihon no iryō-hoken to iryō seido (Japan's health insurance and medical care system). In *Fukushi Kokka 5* (The welfare state 5), ed. Tokyo daigaku shakai kagaku kenkyū-jo. Tokyo: Social Science Research Center, Tokyo Univ.

Sakuma, M. 1978. School health education in Japan. *Social Science and Medicine* 12:551–554.

Steslicke, W. E. 1972. Doctors, patients, and government in modern Japan. *Asian Survey* 12:913–931.

———. 1973. *Doctors in politics*. New York: Praeger.

———. 1982a. Development of health insurance policy in Japan. *Journal of Health Politics, Policy and the Law* 7:197–226.

———. 1982b. Medical care in Japan. *Journal of Ambulatory Care Management* 5:65–77.

———. 1982c. National health policy in Japan. *Bulletin of the Institute for Public Health* 31:1–35.

———. 1984. Medical care for Japan's aging population. *Pacific Affairs* 57:45–52.

Steslicke, W. E., and R. Kimura. 1985. Medical technology for the elderly in Japan. *International Journal of Technology Assessment in Health Care* 1:27–29.

Takemi, T. 1982. *Socialized medicine in Japan*. Tokyo: Japan Medical Association.

Tominaga, K. 1983. Japan's industrial society at critical turn. *The Oriental Economist*, 32–39.

Ward, R. E. 1967. *Japan's political system.* Englewood Cliffs, N.J.: Prentice-Hall.

World Health Organization (WHO). 1980. *Sixth report on the world health situation 1973-1977, part 1.* Geneva: WHO.

———. 1981. *Global strategy for health for all by the year 2000.* Geneva: WHO.

Health Care Providers: Technology, Policy, and Professional Dominance

SUSAN ORPETT LONG

Japanese patients have a wide range of options for obtaining treatment for illness. They may consult a religious specialist or participate in the group therapy of the "new religions." If they prefer a secular cure, they may turn to an herbalist or other folk healer, a specialist in moxibustion or acupuncture, a physician, nurse, or pharmacist. They may elect to treat themselves with home remedies or with over-the-counter medications of natural or synthetic varieties; or, they may do nothing at all. In the broad sense in which most medical anthropologists conceive of a health care system, Japanese health care providers include the shaman, the operator of a hot springs bath, and the dentist.

Yet anyone familiar with modern Japanese society will immediately recognize that all healers are not equal. Biomedicine, introduced by the Portuguese and Spanish in the sixteenth century, has come to occupy a special position in the Japanese health care system. Its legal status, access to governmental and private resources for research and clinical care, and cooptation of certain roles and therapies from traditional medicine all clearly reflect biomedicine's structural dominance.[1] Moreover, within biomedicine there are numerous functionaries, but all are subservient legally and in practice to physicians.

This situation raises three questions: How did biomedical physicians come to dominate the Japanese health care system? What is the nature of that dominance? Will it continue as medicine and society change? I deal with these questions by tracing changes in relations among health providers in two periods. I first consider the introduction of European medicine and the development, through the Tokugawa period (1600–1867), of a corps of biomedical physicians and their relation to the Meiji government's decision in 1868 to promote biomedicine officially. Second, I focus on the period after World War II, which, in parallel to Japan's rapid economic growth, has been characterized by a tremendous expansion of biomedicine and its personnel.

My discussion revolves around two variables, technology and policy. In this context, technology refers to the physical material and techniques applied to the human body for purposes of preventing or curing illness; it does not include the equally important but more abstract aspects of healing such as healer-patient relations or symbolic interpretations of the technology. Although Japan has indigenous medical technology, major technological change has been introduced from other societies, first from China and later from Europe and America. By policy, I mean the plans, decisions, and actions of the central government that affect medical technology and health care providers. Although my original hypothesis was that new technology would result in changing patterns of relationships among healers, I now conclude that the relation is much more complex. As medical sociologist Eliot Freidson (1970, 72) has asserted: "A profession attains and maintains its position by virtue of the protection and patronage of some elite segment of society which has been persuaded that there is some special value in its work. Its position is thus secured by the political and economic influence of the elite which sponsors it."

In the case of Japan, I suggest that the government played and continues to play the role Freidson describes. Government decisions, based on the availability of a certain technology, structure the relationships among health care providers, while at the same time helping to adapt the technology to Japan's specific sociocultural environment.

The Introduction of European Medicine

Medical historians (especially those writing in English) have tended to view the introduction of European medicine as resulting in a dichotomy between "traditional" and "modern" techniques and practices. In the words of one: "The two systems of medicine that came into confrontation were fundamentally divergent. For a millennium, the Japanese practiced traditional medicine, which was completely nonscientific" (Bowers 1980, 157). Accordingly, the decision of the Meiji government to legitimate and support biomedicine becomes, for some, a "triumph" of European "scientific" technology (see, for example, Seaman, who titled his 1906 book *The Real Triumph of Japan*).

Aside from the question of just how scientific sixteenth and seventeenth-century European or Japanese medicine was, the Japanese scene to which European medicine was introduced was far from a unified, static, or unprofessional medical system. Although secular Chinese-style *(kampō)* physicians were established alongside religious specialists as the official health care providers as early as the eighth century, subsequent centuries saw a decline in their influence as Buddhist priest-doctors and folk healers combined the Chinese technology with local custom and practical need. In the fifteenth and sixteenth centuries, however, Neo-Confucian medical theory and practice brought about a revitalization of Chinese-style medicine in Japan, and an elite of secular physicians emerged who served government officials, samurai, and townspeople. The Neo-Confucian influence was systemized and formalized in the sixteenth century by Manase Dōsan into a school known as the *goseiha*.

Even among the elite secular physicians of the Tokugawa period, however, a variety of approaches and methods existed. Another school, the *kohōha*, arose in the seventeenth century and advocated, in opposition to the Neo-Confucians, a return to the classical Chinese medical literature. This school represented a more empirical and simplified practice of medicine which eventually, Otsuka (1976) claims, "Japanized" *goseiha* medicine.[2] Each of these schools had notable followers who published medical books and offered their own versions of Chinese medical theory; it is not clear how these affected the *practice* of most secular doctors. We do know that medical knowledge was obtained in a variety of ways: by attaching oneself formally to a teacher, by studying the classical medical texts (if one were already a Confucian scholar), by independent study, and by unlettered apprenticeship (Fuse 1979, 114). The *goseiha* and *kohōha* movements were undoubtedly most influential in the first and second types of education. We also know that there was no national system of registration and licensure for all physicians, although some official schools did certify their graduates.[3] Many practiced an eclectic medicine, deriving theory and technique from both *goseiha* and *kohōha*, and also from practical experience. (For a discussion of explicit combining by individual scholar-physicians, see Okazaki 1976, 151–152.) Lock (1980, 57) believes that *goseiha* medicine was emphasized in the Kansai region, whereas schools in Kyushu and Edo taught *kohōha* and Western medicine. Writing about the history of medicine in Kyoto, however, Moritani (1978, 100–124) emphasizes the development and practice of *kohōha* and some eclectic schools there. The writings of physicians of both schools, as well as of those using eclectic approaches, were published and available. This, coupled with the fact that patients might try physicians from various schools until they found a successful treatment,[4] leads me to believe that the practitioners were not as far apart in what they actually did as their theoretical classification might lead us to expect.

Although there were undoubtedly strong teacher-pupil loyalties and competition among the various approaches, it is my contention that the overall tone of Tokugawa medicine, at least until the nineteenth century, was one of openness to new ideas, growing empiricism, and syncretism, paralleling trends in eighteenth-century Japanese Confucianism (Craig 1965, 156). Thus, as European medical techniques were gradually introduced, they presented only one more set of options that could be utilized in combination with other technology. In fact, the Japanese scholars and doctors who studied European medicine generally approached it pragmatically. They expressed greatest interest in European surgical technology (methods, medications, etc.), especially in surgery and ophthalmology. Lock (1980, 57) claims that even those drawn to Western surgical technology continued to rely on the Chinese system for internal medicine.[5] Specialists adopted European techniques and established their own "schools" in surgery and ophthalmology (Okazaki 1976, 154). Manase Dōsan, the leader of the *goseiha* movement, was himself influenced by Western medicine and even converted to Christianity in the 1560s or 1570s (Okazaki 1976, 104).

The Official Adoption of Biomedicine

If Western medicine, when first introduced to Japan, added to rather than threatened the existing repertoire of technology, what happened in the last part of the Tokugawa period to polarize Japan's doctors into Western and *kampō* groups by the latter part of the nineteenth century?

First, new technology continued to be brought to Japan. Most authors point to the translation of a German anatomy book, *Anatomische tabellen (Kaitai shinsho),* in 1774 as a turning point in the history of Japanese medicine. Sugita Genpaku and his cotranslators were impressed, after witnessing the dissection of an executed criminal, with the superiority of the book's illustrations over those found in Chinese texts and became determined to make this information available to Japanese doctors and scholars. With the translation of this book, Western medicine was presented as an alternative to the Chinese interpretations, not as a supplement. Moreover, in the last part of the eighteenth century, interest turned toward Western internal medicine, and its drugs were increasingly imported. Most indigenous medications consisted of the crude drug boiled or steeped in hot water (infusions and decoctions, while alcohol-based fluid extracts and aromatics were avoided), which accorded with Japanese tradition (Okazaki 1976, 180). Otsuka notes that when the first work on Western internal medicine was published in 1793 it contained a preface by a famous physician-official; this preface was removed from the second edition, "probably because younger practitioners of *kampō* and *Rampō*[6] stood against such a cooperative—or, from another point of view, conciliatory—attitude" (Otsuka 1976, 333). The greatest change in technology may have been the introduction of public health measures to combat contagious disease, particularly the introduction of the live smallpox vaccination in 1824 and 1849 (see Otsuka 1976, 334).

These technological innovations were only indirectly responsible for the later dominance of biomedical physicians, however. The intermediate step was the obtaining of government sponsorship. From 1739, when the government sent two scholar-officials to Nagasaki to study Dutch, the attitude of government might be characterized as active tolerance of Western medicine. This was the beginning of the avid translation of Dutch scientific books, although it is unlikely that at this point many outside the intelligentsia were affected. By the first half of the nineteenth century, doctors who had studied with the Dutch at Nagasaki established their own private medical schools, and biomedicine was included in the curriculum of at least some official *han* schools. Philipp Franz Balthasar Von Siebold, a physician from a prominent German medical family, served from 1823 to 1828 at the Dutch station. He received permission to see patients in Nagasaki rather than being restricted to Dejima (the island where all foreigners were required at that time to reside) and later built a medical school on the outskirts of Nagasaki, where he gave clinical lectures on internal medicine as well as surgery.

There was as yet no organized opposition on the part of the Chinese-style practitioners, although by the 1840s a number of practicing physicians identified themselves as "Western medical" specialists (Moritani 1978, 125). However, the ailing economic and social position of the Edo government did provide the opportunity for one last display of power for at least one school, the Taki, that combined elements of *kohōha* and *goseiha* (Okazaki 1976, 151). The Taki family had come to control the government's Medical Bureau and served as personal physicians to the shogun. When the government decided that, in order to bolster its own position, it was necessary to rid itself of foreign influence,[7] the Takis took advantage of the new policy to strengthen their own control over medical theory and practice. The government outlawed the use of Dutch words in advertising medicines, restricted publication of Dutch books, supervised their importation and sale, and subjected all publications of Dutch medical translations to the censorship of the Taki-controlled Medical Bureau. Medical books published between 1840 and 1853 were those that supported the Takis' own approach (Sugaya 1976, 4; Kawakami 1977, 90).

Dutch medicine nevertheless continued to be practiced. The decision to end the 200-year-old closed-country *(sakoku)* system and reopen Japan in the face of Western pressure in the 1850s caused a complete turn around in the official attitude toward foreign technology. The government was now convinced that the only way to remain sovereign was to adopt foreign technology, particularly military technology. The internal warfare that characterized the end of the Tokugawa and early Meiji periods intensified an interest in surgical treatment. In 1857 the Edo government requested that the Dutch send a military surgeon to train Japanese physicians; as a result, J. L. C. Pompe van Meedervort was allowed to establish a school in Nagasaki with a full biomedical curriculum, including instruction in the basic sciences. Moreover, an official government physician, Matsumoto Ryōjun, requested and received permission to study there and assist in setting up the new school, despite the fact that restrictions of foreign study remained in effect (Bowers 1970, 178).

The new government policy toward foreign technology also allowed official support of public health measures such as vaccinations. In 1858 Dutch-style doctors in Edo established the Vaccination Institute as a private institution funded by subscription. "Although it used the name 'Vaccination Institute,' it served at the same time to promote Western medicine" (Kawakami 1977, 88). Within several years the institute received a government subsidy (Bowers 1970, 195). The government also decided to support a surgical hospital in Edo (Fuse 1979, 133) as well as Pompe's medical school, laboratories, and hospital in Nagasaki. Several authors (for example, Okazaki 1976, 213; Bowers 1970, 189) see a direct relation between Pompe's efforts in controlling a cholera epidemic and his receiving government funds, which had been requested several years previously. The final blow to the power of the Chinese-style doctors came in 1858 when they failed to cure the ailing shogun. Dutch-style physicians were then called in to serve as court physicians, providing de facto recognition of the change in governmental attitude.

Thus, the Tokugawa government, ten years before the Meiji Restoration, had already adopted a policy of promoting biomedicine. The positive attitude toward Western biomedicine was partly a response to Western technology as it was displayed by European and American military might in the 1850s. It was also in many ways a continuation of a trend of growing interest in biomedical technology as it was gradually introduced and proven useful in the Japanese context. Chinese-style physicians such as the Takis did not react until they were sufficiently threatened by government interest in and support of biomedicine.

The Meiji government took the final steps in assuring the dominant position of biomedicine. The government decided to support biomedical education and research institutes based on the German system;[8] it founded public biomedical hospitals and began a national system of physician licensure. Proclamations of 1875 and 1883 restricted the practice of Chinese-style medicine to those holding biomedical degrees, thus subordinating *kampō* to the biomedical system. Practitioners of massage and acupuncture had to be licensed as well, and their practice was limited by law so that they were no threat to physicians. It was in this period that the term *kampō* first came to be used, thus indicating the polarization of biomedicine and Chinese-style medicine. In reaction, *kampō* physicians organized themselves for purposes of education and research and for political reasons. From the second session of the newly established Diet (1891), the *kampō* physicians' association tried to legislate changes in licensure and registration. A bill was finally brought to a vote in 1895 and defeated. Over 63 percent of Japanese doctors at this time still had no training in biomedicine (Fuse 1979, 146).[9]

How was it that biomedicine had such strong support in government circles? One factor was the infatuation of Meiji leaders with Western technology in general. Medicine was a small but highly visible part of their dramatic effort to modernize quickly and so avoid colonization. Biomedicine as a social institution also gained strength in part through interbureaucratic rivalries and rivalry between the Diet and the bureaucracy (see Bartholomew 1982). The effect was that "Meiji doctors, ordered by the government to discard traditional medical practices and ideas and switch to Western medicine, without regard for the ruin of *kampō* physicians, became an intelligensia, an elite bearing one part of the burden of national prosperity" (Fuse 1979, 211).

A second factor was that many of the people who played leadership roles in and out of the government had studied at the Tokugawa-period schools of Dutch learning, receiving instruction directly from the foreigners at Nagasaki and later from their followers in Edo, Kyoto, and Osaka.[10] As students of Dutch learning, they not only favored adoption of Western technology, but had developed intense loyalties to teachers and classmates.

There were, however, important continuities in the nature of medical practice from the Tokugawa to the Meiji period. Although the government insisted on westernization, as in the previous period, an elite of physicians received public support, whereas most of the system remained private as in Tokugawa times. Payment for medications prescribed by physicians continued to be the responsibility of patients or their families. Medicine in both Tokugawa and Meiji Japan was a full-time male occupation, and a practitioner in both periods could earn a living through relatively autonomous medical practice (Fuse 1979; Bartholomew 1982). Furthermore, Bartholomew's research on the formation of the Meiji scientific community shows that the social class background of medical practitioners in the early Meiji period was similar to that of recruits in the last half of the Tokugawa period. In his sample of 189 scientists, 101 had physician-fathers and 75 of these were *kampō* physicians (1980, 69). Bartholomew concludes that:

> When the sons of Chinese-style physicians realized the possibilities of careers in modern chemistry or biomedical science, they entered those fields as circumstances allowed with little or no thought to their intellectual incompatibility with Chinese-style medicine. The modern biomedical science tradition in particular developed rapidly in post-Restoration Japan precisely because it was able to exploit not only the *presence* of Chinese medicine but because it could build on its institutional patterns—autonomy, occupational base, rigorous training and certification programs—which had already come into existence during the Tokugawa period. (1980, 72)

Medicine, now limited to biomedicine, must have been an attractive career in the Meiji period, even more so than today. It meant, for the practitioner, financial security and prestige as a healer and as a "modern"; it also afforded opportunities for a high level of intellectual attainment and, for a few, study abroad, a university position, or government employment. Rather than having to organize to fight for a favored role in the new society, biomedical physicians were selected by the government for sponsorship; it was not until 1875 that for academic and political purposes, the first organization for biomedical physicians was founded. Prefectural governments encouraged the formation of medical associations from 1886 on as a way of influencing individual physicians (Kawakami 1977, 231–232). Various specialty groups and academic medical societies were also founded in the latter part of the Meiji period. The Japan Medical Association (Dai Nippon Ikai), with membership limited to licensed practitioners, was founded in 1893 in the midst of the Diet debate about licensure for Chinese-style doctors.

Professional Organization Today

Although great progress has been made since the 1920s in universalizing access to care and in developing indirect methods of payment, the structure of the medical profession has changed little from Meiji or even Tokugawa times. Meiji prohibitions against practicing *kampō* without a biomedical license remain in effect. The recent "*kampō* boom" of popular interest in herbal medications, which has been sparked or encouraged by biomedical pharmaceutical companies, has not been to the benefit of *kampō*. The result of the "boom" has been the inclusion of some *kampō* medications among those eligible for insurance reimbursement, and thus their widespread use and misuse by biomedical physicians with little knowledge of *kampō* theory or practice (Lock 1984). In order to become licensed, practitioners of massage and acupuncture must complete prescribed courses of study structurally similar to those of biomedical paraprofessional workers such as nurses. Thus, despite the negative publicity about synthetic drugs and their prescribers, the "*kampō* boom" has, if anything, only further subordinated *kampō* to biomedicine.

The government continues to directly support only a minority of physicians. For the most part, the system still relies on "*machi-isha,*" private practitioners of the common people, as in Tokugawa times. Although less than half of Japanese physicians are in private practice, these private practitioners account for over 90 percent of primary care clinics and 75 percent of hospitals (Hashimoto 1978a, 23).

Professors, assistant professors, and lecturers at the prestigious national university medical schools, administrative and staff doctors at nationally supported hospitals, as well as a small number of physicians engaged in full-time research constitute the national government-employed group. This group has counterparts at prefectural and local levels, but with somewhat less prestige. These salaried physicians may historically be most similar to the retained doctors of the Tokugawa government and daimyo. Unlike the Meiji professors, who spent the majority of their time seeing private patients, probably in order to support themselves (see Bartholomew n.d.), contemporary public hospital and university physicians rarely establish their own private practices or spend more than a small amount of their time on professional pursuits outside of the hospital or university that is their major employer.

Salaried doctors may be divided into various groups. Some are employed by the Ministry of Education, some by the Ministry of Health and Welfare, and some by prefectural and local governments. A salaried physician may be a clinician or a researcher or, as is most common in university settings, may fill both roles. Physicians are also divided by their specialities within biomedicine. Overall, the interests and organizations of salaried doctors differ from those of private practitioners.

As entrepreneurs, private practitioners must concern themselves to a greater extent than do their salaried counterparts with satisfying their patients' expectations. In order to be paid they must deal with the demands and the red tape of the complex insurance system. As in any business, they need to pay their employees and other overhead costs. These physicians have specialty and interest groups that provide mutual support at the local level. Nationally, their common interests are represented by the Japan Medical Association.[11]

The media and the public in Japan view the JMA as a powerful influence on the government. It attempts to influence policy mainly through the bureaucracy, having formal representation on a number of advisory boards such as the Social Security System Council, the Medical Fee Payment Fund, and the Social Insurance Council. It lobbies for favorable policy decisions and has even sponsored nationwide work stoppages. The JMA also attempts to influence policy indirectly through support of physicians or other sympathetic candidates for political office and through "public education" campaigns (Steslicke 1973).

On the other hand, pressures directed in the reverse direction, at individual practitioners, constitute an equally significant aspect of government-physician relations. I have already pointed out that biomedical physicians' groups were formed in the Meiji period at the encouragement of the government. In 1961, despite opposition to various aspects of the program from many private practitioners and the JMA, the government established a universal insurance system. Opposition from business and labor has foiled JMA attempts since then to unify and rationalize this system.

Private practitioners, through the JMA, are given some voice in determining legal regulations governing their practices and in fixing the insurance reimbursement schedule on which their livelihood depends, but they are far from having the power to determine policy. As long as it cannot, or will not, nationalize the medical system fully, the government must be willing to keep private physicians relatively satisfied. But although the government must accommodate private practitioners, it is not willing to withdraw its control. Private as well as salaried physicians must bow to overall government policy that determines to a large extent the nature of their work and their daily routines. The financial structure of the system virtually eliminates the practice of preventive medicine or patient education and encourages physicians to see large numbers of patients (whose visits are consequently brief) and the dispensing of large amounts of medication. As the intermediary between government and private practitioner, the JMA can, by vetoing clinic locations, refusing to file insurance forms, and so on, at the local level, make practice difficult or impossible for private practitioners who oppose it (Nomura 1976). It thus has a role in enforcing government policy as well as in shaping it.

Physician Dominance in an Age of High-Technology Medicine

The spectacular growth of the field of medicine (and the medicalization of many aspects of society) experienced in the United States since World War II has had its counterpart in Japan. Kawakami (1977, 525) notes that the technological revolution in medicine has meant new synthetic pharmaceuticals, the development of antibiotics, progress in surgery, and reliance on clinical laboratory tests and X rays. He suggests that these new elements of biomedicine have created changes in hospital construction and management, particularly the inclusion of a central laboratory and changes in surgical facilities. The new technology increasingly replaces the one-to-one doctor-patient relationship with medical care provided by a health care team.

As in the United States, costs have also risen dramatically. As the Japanese government concentrated on policies of high economic growth in the 1950s and 1960s, some attention was given to public health, particularly to the eradication of tuberculosis and other infectious diseases. The government pieced together a complex universal insurance program, which went into effect in 1961. However, as late as 1970, only 3.32 percent of Japan's GNP was spent on medical care; the government came under increasing attack in the late 1960s and 1970s for neglecting social services and for actually promoting medical problems such as pollution-related disease through its high-growth policy. In 1973 a program for medical care for the elderly went into effect and a program of catastrophic insurance began. By 1980 the cost of medical care constituted over 5 percent of Japan's GNP, although the government's share of that cost remained fairly constant between the mid-1960s and 1980 (see table 1).

The changes in medical technology have created new roles for health workers. In addition to the physicians, nurses, and pharmacists found before World War II, there are now nutritionists, speech therapists, artificial limb technicians, physical therapists, cytology technicians, medical photographers, and clinical engineers. Endoscopic technicians have their own professional organization of 71,000 members (*Byōin* 1981). Physicists also work with radiologists, and audiologists help otolaryngologists.

Not only has the variety of health providers increased, but the number of health workers has risen dramatically both in absolute terms and relative to population size (see table 2). Only among midwives has a decrease occurred, a result of physicians taking over prenatal and childbirth care. Moreover, there seems to be a trend toward an increasing proportion of

Table 1. Japanese Medical Costs as Percentage of GNP

Year	GNP	Direct Public Expense as Percentage of Medical Costs
1955	2.69	
1960	2.53	
1965	3.35	12.6*
1970	3.32	11.3
1975	4.27	13.1
1980	5.01	12.3

Sources: Ministry of Health and Welfare statistics from Kōsei Tōkei Kyōkai 1982, 248, 249) and Nihon Ishikai (1977, 395).
* 1966 figure.

health providers employed by hospitals. In 1970, 37 percent of physicians worked as salaried employees; by 1980 this figure had increased to 48 percent (Nihon Ishikai 1977, 396; Kōsei Tōkei Kyōkai 1982, 210). Among nurses, the proportion of hospital-employed has risen for registered nurses and for nurse-midwives (as opposed to private practice for the latter) and has decreased slightly for practical nurses (Kōseishō 1982, 2–7). The great increase among technicians reflects occupations which are hospital based: 72 percent for X ray and radiology, 83 percent for laboratory (as opposed to physicians, public health nurses, or pharmacists) (statistics from Kōsei Tōkei Kyōkai 1982, 210–214).

The increase in the variety and numbers of biomedical health workers suggests that major changes are occurring in relations among health providers and, as medicine has become more bureaucratic, between providers and patients. Some writers expect that paramedical workers will become more assertive and that the dominance of physicians will be lessened. They claim that medical education does not provide physicians with the knowledge of how to utilize the new technology (Tani 1973, 103), and physicians thus become more dependent upon the technicians they are supposed to supervise (Ishihara 1981). Paramedicals, operating through medical labor unions organized after World War II, have demanded better wages and working conditions (the most noticeable instance was in 1960, during a nationwide hospital strike) (see Kawakami 1977, 525–529).

Table 2. Increase in Health Care Workers

	1960	1970	Increase from 1960	1980	Increase from 1970
Physician	103,131	118,990	15	148,815	25
Pharmacist	60,257	79,393	32	116,656	47
Public health nurse	13,010	14,007	8	17,957	28
Midwife	55,436	31,559	−43	27,388	−13
Registered nurse	105,800	139,229	32	261,613	88
Practical nurse	70,065	164,464	135	257,219	56
Laboratory technician	9,984[a]	12,622	26	17,963[b]	42
X-ray and radiology technician	8,588	15,984	86	39,956[b]	150
Total population in 1,000 persons	94,302	104,665	11	117,060	12

Sources: Ministry of Health and Welfare statistics from Hashimoto (1978b, 534) and Kōsei Tōkei Kyōkai (1982, 210).
[a] 1965 figure.
[b] 1978 figure.

Despite the trends of change discussed above, including the creation and aggressiveness of medical labor unions, several factors mitigate against any substantial alteration in the physicians' role of dominance in the medical system. All of these factors may be traced, at least in part, to the government's sponsorship of their dominance. The most obvious example is that laws relating to paramedical workers (including practitioners of acupuncture and massage) state explicitly that the medical activities of these workers are limited to those under the direction or direct orders of physicians. Judging from the comments of an official of the Ministry of Health and Welfare, these limitations are interpreted quite literally. When asked about the best personnel to deal with new medical technology, this official discussed the need to treat each case separately according to the medical knowledge and skill required for it. As far as hearing tests, artificial dialysis, pacemakers, and the like are concerned, "at the present time, all of these techniques can be considered most appropriately performed by a physician or a nurse assisting him" (*Byōin* 1981, 757). Although the ministry recognizes that its conservative policies are detrimental to both the development of an adequate supply and the quality of paramedical workers, it remains unwilling to grant them greater autonomy. Hashimoto Masami, former head of the Department of Public Health Practice within the Ministry of Health and Welfare, expressed the ministry's ambivalent attitude.

> It is apparent that recent trends and changing patterns in health caused by rapid changes in socio-economic and socio-biological conditions require the development of various new types of health personnel.
> Under the present situation in Japan, however, . . . well planned governmental efforts for the improvement of the education and training methods and the social status of these health personnel should be promoted. The strengthening and effective training of teaching staff, the establishment of continuing education systems, a deepening understanding with the medical professions on the problem seem to be important. At the same time, selected new types of health disciplines must be developed cautiously. (Hashimoto 1978b, 538)

Deference shown to physicians by paramedical workers may be traced in part to the influence of Japanese patterns of interpersonal behavior. Expectations surrounding male-female interaction are important. Over 90 percent of physicians are men, women doctors being concentrated in a few specialties such as opthalmology and pediatrics. By contrast, women usually fill subordinate roles. Fifty-five percent of pharmacists and 97 percent of nurses are women (Kōseishō 1982, 10–11; Kōsei Tōkei Kyōkai 1982, 211, 212). Behavior patterns from outside the work setting, such as those between husbands and wives, may easily be transferred to the medical context (Long 1984).

The length and type of education most paramedical workers require differ greatly from the training of physicians in medical school and postgraduate programs. Most nurses and many other paramedical workers receive their training at special vocational schools that are generally considered inferior to college and university programs in terms of faculties, facilities, and educational curricula. A few occupations, such as pharmacy, require baccalaureate degrees, but most require only graduation from junior colleges. Although the government cannot dictate the ways in which sex roles and educational attainment should affect social status or interpersonal relations, the perpetuation of the social gap between physicians and other health workers must be considered an indirect result of government educational and licensing requirements, laws relating to working conditions, and wage structure.

Physician dominance is also indirectly maintained through laws regulating hospital organization. Prewar hospitals were characterized by what Ishihara (1981) calls "vertical" organization, in which a paramedical worker was attached to one or another specialty department headed by a physician. During the postwar occupation, the Allied forces attempted to democratize the medical system by creating the "horizontal" organization found in American hospitals, in which pharmacy, nursing service, laboratory, and so on each have a separate administrative unit with a nonphysician head. This reform did not take hold in most university hospitals in Japan. Private hospitals, which the government had in the past encouraged to proliferate, remain under the firm control of their entrepreneurial physician founders. Even in the large public hospitals where there is "horizontal" organization, the official structure appears to have had little impact at the behavioral level, and paramedical workers continue to believe they are working for a specialty department or for a doctor. Legally, a hospital director must be a physician, so that even in the most horizontal of structures, paramedical departments remain subordinate.

A final policy maintaining the physicians' dominance of the medical system has been the government's attempt to increase the physician-to-population ratio to 150 per 100,000 population by 1985 (the 1980 ratio was 141 per 100,000 population [Kōsei Tōkei Kyōkai 1982, 214]). The government thus promoted the establishment of numerous new medical schools (mostly private) in the 1960s and 1970s, many of which are considered inferior to the public (especially national) university medical schools. This expansion has raised total annual enrollment at all medical schools from 2,840 students in 1960 to 8,260 students in 1980 (Kōsei Tōkei Kyōkai 1982, 215).

This policy has several consequences. First, by greatly expanding the size of the occupational group, it makes physicians less of an elite group vis-à-vis other interest groups attempting to influence policy. Theoretically, if all the new graduates were to go into private practice, competition for patients would increase and incomes of physicians would decline. But within the public medical system, ironically, the effect has been to maintain the positions of those in power. Large numbers of young physicians in university and public sector hospitals mean that more experienced doctors can delegate tasks to them (as apprentices) rather than having to rely on paramedicals. Even though Japanese physicians are highly specialized in their medical training and practice, because of their large numbers many of them will remain generalists in both tasks and responsibilities. Young doctors often perform work that in the United States would be assigned to nurses (for example, history taking in outpatient clinics) and laboratory personnel, thus reducing the effect of the shortage of paramedical workers.

Large numbers of young doctors also strengthen the *ikyoku* system (see Long 1980, 112–123, 158–160), the "feudal" hierarchy of doctors under a single departmental professor that has been a feature of biomedical education and research since the Meiji government decided to adopt many aspects of the German model of Western medicine. In this system, a young physician relies on his professor for introductions to employment opportunities. In exchange for some loss of autonomy in these decisions, the young doctor, by maintaining good relations with his professor, assures receptivity to referrals of private patients, access to new developments in his field, and sometimes access to research facilities, any of which might help to advance his career. The professor, for his part, needs to cultivate good relations with administrator-physicians at hospitals and with private practitioners in the area to obtain political and financial support, including employment for the young doctors in his department.

During the war years the government decided to increase rapidly the number of physicians and so promoted shortened courses at local governmental and private medical schools. When the war ended, many young doctors turned to the university medical departments for further education and for help in obtaining employment, thus fostering the continuation of the hierarchy they had known earlier. Despite attempts to democratize medical schools after World War II, this hierarchic system was particularly strong in the 1950s and 1960s.

Several changes began to threaten the *ikyoku* system in the 1960s. Although the system was the target of a revolt by medical students and interns in the late sixties, the success of the revolt seems to have stemmed from socioeconomic and technical changes rather than mere protest against the educational system. Although the number of physicians had increased, government policy, especially the establishment of the universal insurance system, had created a *relative* shortage. Hospitals competed for physicians, approaching them directly rather than through their professors and offering higher salaries than in the past. At the same time, specialized, high-technology medicine made general private practice more expensive and less prestigious, and thus a less desirable career option while higher hospital salaries created a financially viable alternative, thus somewhat relieving the physician shortage in public hospitals. For both of these reasons hospital employment became a viable alternative.

In recent years, as economic growth has slowed, so also has the increase in the number of hospital beds (Kōsei Tōkei Kyōkai 1982, 204). The need for expensive equipment and changes in tax laws have made it more difficult to enter private practice, as has pressure from local medical associations. Thus, an increase in young physicians comes at a time of changing employment and career opportunities. This circumstance seems to have the effect of restrengthening the power of professors, administrator-physicians, and others who are at the top of the medical hierarchy.

Conclusion

By examining the Japanese medical system in two periods, I have attempted to explore and explain the relationship between technological change and professional dominance. The introduction of Western medicine, which occurred gradually over a period of three hundred years, culminated in 1868 with the government's declaration of support for a German-style medical system. This declaration reflects what Lee (1982) calls the "structural superiority" that Western medicine had achieved. Inroads were also made in expanding its "functional strength," the distribution and utilization of Western medicine so as to increase its impact on the society as a whole. Unlike Lee's Chinese examples, however, these changes did not come about through professional organization in Japan; rather, the government sponsored such changes in the course of promoting its own interests. It was not, therefore, the introduction of biomedical technology itself that brought about the dominance of biomedical physicians. Certainly, that technology had first to be made available (by, among other things, overcoming the language barrier) and then shown to be effective. But there were other factors of equal importance in determining government policy, in particular, the economic and social weakness of the late Tokugawa government and the threat to Japanese sovereignty posed by the European military powers. Technology plus politics determined the shape of the Meiji medical system.

In the period since World War II, biomedicine's functional strength was assured by economic growth (see Lee 1982) and the establishment of a universal health insurance system. As a result of worldwide trends in biomedicine, technological innovations have occurred at a rapid rate, and the Japanese government has pursued a policy of supporting what I call "high-technology medicine." Such technology could curb the dominance of the system by physicians who are unable to control the technology and who, as a result, become only one part of a more specialized division of labor in a bureaucratic setting. However, while accepting or even encouraging technological change, the government has been cautious about altering the social structure of the medical system. Its policies have maintained the subordinate status of paramedical workers and the power of physicians in high-level university and hospital positions. Thus, while in the earlier period technological change led to sociocultural change through government support, more recent changes in the nature of medical technology have had only limited impact in this regard.

The circumstances described above have several implications for our broader understanding of the relationship between technological and sociocultural change. First, it appears that there is no direct relationship in which technology determines social structure. In neither of the periods I have discussed did the Japanese government create policy merely in reaction to changes in available medical technology. Rather, it investigated the technology, studied its possible consequences, and attempted to direct the speed of its introduction and to control its use. Thus, to understand the Japanese medical scene, we need microlevel political and socio-logical studies that treat government officials and professionals as well as patients as active decision makers. Such research would clarify the abstract concepts of "government" and "profession" by revealing the relationships among individuals with different areas of expertise and the procedures by which they make decisions. This would lead to a fuller understanding of the specific conditions under which technical change will lead to changes in social structure.

The second implication of this study is that the result of decision making cannot be viewed as blind copying, of which the Japanese have often been accused. The Japanese version of biomedicine today has certainly been greatly influenced by the seventeenth and eighteenth-century Dutch, nineteenth-century German, and twentieth-century American medical systems that served as its models. But from the beginning, when Japanese physicians concentrated on European surgical techniques, the "borrowing" was selective. Bartholomew (1974) points to several important differences between Meiji medicine and its German model. Despite the similarity in the technology of biomedicine in Japan and the United States today, there are notable differences in the structure of their systems, in the organization of their medical professions, and in relations among their health care workers. Differences, as Ben-David has written of scientific activity in general, do not arise because social values determine the content (here, technology) of science. But two types of conditions influence differences in the nature of scientific activity: "the changing constellation of social values and interests among populations as a whole which channeled the motivation of people to support, believe, or engage in science . . . [and] the organization of scientific work" (Ben-David 1971, 169).

In Japan the government has played a direct role in creating both of these conditions, but it has done so by including elements of the past as well as imported technology. My examination shows continuities in the role of the physician as a "professional," the dependence on private practice, the cultural interpretations of sex roles and educational background that influence social ranking, and the importance of government-physician relations. Policy, then, may be viewed as a factor intervening between technology and social structure, helping to adapt technology to a specific sociocultural environment. I would therefore question the assumptions of those who argue for an eventual convergence of Japanese and Western social systems. Careful investigation of the medical system of Japan does not show that the adoption of foreign technology leads automatically to changes in social structure. Rather, the technology and social structure of Japan's medical system have both faced the scrutiny of people in positions of power.

Notes

In addition to published sources on the history of medicine in Japan and on the current medical system, many of the ideas presented in this study result from my year's observation in 1977–1978 of the Japanese medical system and from interviews and discussions with numerous biomedical health care providers. I am grateful to my fellow panelists at the 1983 meeting of the American Anthropological Association, at which this paper was initially presented, and to James Bartholomew and David Plath for their comments and suggestions.

1. For example, midwifery, a folk healer role, now requires a special degree and is legally classified with nursing. For a discussion of how *kampō* physicians (specialists in the prescription of herbal medicine) must have biomedical licenses and the recent inclusion of certain herbal medication in the insurance system, see Lock 1980 and 1984.

2. Lock (1980) follows Otsuka (1976) in characterizing the return to the classical Chinese text (A.D. 200) the *Shang han lun* (A treatise on fevers) as a uniquely Japanese development. On the other hand Okazaki (1976, 147) claims that a call for a return to the classics arose in Ch'ing China. Although this interesting question needs to be resolved, it is only a side issue to the thrust of my argument here.

3. Some *han,* or feudal domains, sponsored medical schools and certification for that *han.*

4. I base this assumption on stories about a healer being called in after an earlier attempt by another healer has failed to bring results (see, for example, Okazaki 1976, 148) and my observations of contemporary health-seeking behavior in Japan.

5. This may be due in part to the lack of knowledge of European internal medicine in the early Tokugawa period.

6. *Rampō* literally means "Dutch medicine." The term contrasts the Dutch-German style of Western medicine of Tokugawa with both the Sino-Japanese and the Southern European style introduced earlier.

7. I here follow the argument that it was primarily the government's recognition of its own weakness that led to these policies. In medicine, however, an additional factor was present. Siebold, a German physician employed by the Dutch at Dejima, had been caught smuggling a map of Japan and other contraband out of the country in 1828. Siebold had been particularly active both in teaching Western medicine and in learning about Japan and had become highly

respected. This incident may have increased the government's xenophobia in the 1830s (Bowers 1970, 92–126; Okazaki 1976, 198–210).

8. The Japanese government considered other models of biomedicines, in particular the more public-health-oriented British system, but decided in favor of the German system. The prestige of German medicine in Europe, especially the spectacular advances in the bacteriology of the late nineteenth century (see Bartholomew 1974, 1982) and the familiarity with German texts, teachers, and so on, from Tokugawa "Dutch medicine" seem to have been important factors in this decision (see Bowers 1980).

9. Fuse (1979, 146) provides the following breakdown for 1899:

Kampō physicians		24,720
Biomedical physicians		14,056
University graduates	1,462	
Medical school graduates	3,301	
Foreign graduates or		
licensure by examination	7,916	
Public officials or teachers		1,377
Unknown		438
Total		39,214

10. Fukuzawa Yukichi, a student of Ōgata Kōan, is perhaps the best-known example. For discussions of the role of physicians as modernizers in other Asian nations, see Silcock 1977 and Madan 1980.

11. Salaried physicians can and do join the Japan Medical Association, but the association is broken down into separate sections. According to Nakano (1976, 108–109), 72 percent of Japan's physicians are members, broken down as follows:

Section A—private practitioners	73%
Section B—employed clinical physicians	25%
Section C—university or research	
institute staff	2%

In my experience, physicians join Sections B and C because their hospital automatically pays their dues and/or, in the case of administrator-physicians, for political reasons.

References

Bartholomew, J. R. 1974. Japanese culture and the problem of modern science. In *Science and values,* ed. A. Thackray and E. Mendelsohn. New York: Humanities Press.
———. 1980. The Japanese scientific community in formation, 1870–1920. In

Science in modern East Asia, vol. 1, ed. L. A. Schneider. Buffalo: State Univ. of New York, *Journal of Asian Affairs* 5(1).

————. 1982. Science, bureaucracy, and freedom in Meiji and Taishō Japan. In *Conflict in modern Japanese history*, ed. T. Najita and J. V. Koschmann. Princeton: Princeton Univ. Press.

————. N.d. The formation of science in Japan. Forthcoming.

Ben-David, J. 1971. *The scientist's role in society*. Englewood Cliffs, N.J.: Prentice-Hall.

Bowers, J. Z. 1970. *Western medical pioneers in feudal Japan*. Baltimore: Johns Hopkins Univ. Press.

————. 1980. *When the twain meet*. Baltimore: Johns Hopkins Univ. Press.

Byōin. 1981. *Paramedikaru bumon no kakudai* (The expansion of the paramedical section). Special Issue, 40(9).

Craig, A. 1965. Science and Confucianism in Tokugawa Japan. In *Changing Japanese attitudes toward modernization,* ed. M. B. Jansen. Princeton: Princeton Univ. Press.

Freidson, E. 1970. *Profession of medicine*. New York: Dodd, Mead, and Co.

Fuse, S. 1979. *Ishi no rekishi* (The history of physicians). Tokyo: Chūō Kōronsha.

Hashimoto, M. 1978a. Health and the medical system in Japan. MS.

————. 1978b. The professional education and training of non-medical health personnel in Japan. *Social Science and Medicine* 12A:533–538.

Ishihara, S. 1981. *Byōin sōshiki ni okeru paramedikaru bumon no arikata* (The paramedical section in hospital organization). *Byōin* 40:738–742.

Kawakami, T. 1977. *Gendai Nihon iryōshi* (The history of modern Japanese medicine). 8th ed. Tokyo: Chikuma Shobō.

Kōseishō Imukyoku Kangoka Kanshū. 1982. *Shōwa 57 kango kankei tōkei shiryō shū* (1982 statistical data related to nursing). Tokyo: Nihon Kango Kyōkai Shuppankai.

Kōsei Tōkei Kyōkai. 1982. Kokumin eisei no dōkō (Trends in national public health). Special Issue, *Kōsei no Shihyō*, 29(9).

Lee, R. P. L. 1982. Comparative studies of health care systems. *Social Science and Medicine* 16:629–642.

Lock, M. 1980. *East Asian medicine in urban Japan*. Berkeley and Los Angeles: Univ. of California Press.

————. 1984. Licorice in leviathan. The medicalization of care for the Japanese Elderly. *Culture, Medicine and Psychiatry* 8:121–139.

Long, S. O. 1980. Fame, fortune, and friends. Ph.D. diss. University of Illinois, Urbana.

————. 1984. The sociocultural context of nursing in Japan. *Culture, Medicine and Psychiatry* 8:141–164.

Madan, T. N., ed. 1980. *Doctors and society*. Ghaziabad, U.P., India: Vikas.

Moritani, K. 1978. *Miyako ishi no rekishi* (The history of Kyoto physicians). Tokyo: Kodansha.

Nakano, H. 1976. *Gendai Nihon no ishi* (Modern Japanese physicians). Tokyo: Nikkei Shinsho.

Nihon Ishikai. 1977. *Kokumin iryō nenkan* (People's medical yearbook). Tokyo: Shinshūsha.

Nomura, T. 1976. *Nihon Ishikai* (The Japan Medical Association). Tokyo: Keisō Shobō.

Okazaki, K. 1976. *Kusuri no rekishi* (The history of medicine). Tokyo: Kodansha.

Otsuka, Y. 1976. Chinese traditional medicine in Japan. In *Asian Medical Systems,* ed. C. Leslie. Berkeley and Los Angeles: Univ. of California Press.

Seaman, L. L. 1906. *The real triumph of Japan.* New York: D. Appleton and Co.

Silcock, T. H., ed. 1977. *Professional structure in Southeast Asia.* Canberra: Australian National Univ.

Steslicke, W. E. 1973. *Doctors in politics.* New York: Praeger.

Sugaya, A. 1976. *Nihon iryō seido shi* (The history of the Japanese medical system). Tokyo: Hara Shobō.

Tani, M. 1973. *Jūjishatachi no ariyō* (Health care workers). In *Iryō o sasaeru hito-bito* (The people who maintain the medical system), ed. Asahi Shimbunsha. Tokyo: Asahi Shimbunsha.

Care of the Aged in Japan

Christie W. Kiefer

Technology and the "Ugly Decline"

The pursuit of scientific and technological progress has been, by practically any measure, Japan's forte in this century. It is a pursuit that carries heavy costs in any society, but most consider it worth those costs because it seems to bring some image of a satisfying life closer to reality for the great majority of people. The ingredients of this satisfying life differ in detail from culture to culture and person to person, but fundamentally they include increased control over the conditions of one's life or at least greater freedom from the bonds of poverty, illness, and arbitrary rule. It is a great irony, then, that any technologically advanced society brings to the lives of a majority of its people a long period of powerlessness, illness, and confinement. No advanced culture has yet resisted the power of technology to postpone death; yet none has found a way to guarantee freedom and dignity to even a sizeable minority of the resulting masses of disabled, frail, and terminally ill.

It becomes more and more likely that what the Japanese call the "ugly decline" *(hen na kakō)* will be a larger and larger share of each life. Yet there is no simple way to alter this process. Once a society has, one, the technological means to delay death for a substantial population, two, the political means to provide popular access to this technology, and three, an information industry that can quickly measure and disseminate the effects of one and two on mass longevity, then government will begin to use longevity itself as one measure of its strength and economic effectiveness. It will have entered what David Plath has called "the aging Olympics." There is a vicious economic circle in this process, which the recent history of Japan illustrates admirably.

As longevity increases, society at first applauds, pouring resources (and prestige) into the health care sector (see Lock and Long, this volume). At a later point the growing misery of the old unwell becomes apparent, but the first step cannot be reversed. Society must take a greater role in health care because of the economic dependency of this new "health problem" population. Later, I will discuss some examples of this process. The "ugly decline" is always bought at an ever higher cost to society as a whole, a cost not only in dollars but in the labor and anxiety of those, mostly wrinkled and grey themselves, who watch over that decline and try to lighten its oppression.

Aging Japan

Because Japan industrialized late, fast, and thoroughly, the aging of Japanese society has also been sudden and disruptive. English-language reports of this phenomenon now span ten years (Plath 1972, 1973, 1980, 1983; Sparks 1973, 1975; Kinoshita 1981; D. Maeda 1983; Steslicke 1984), and a few statistics will convey its scope.

> The proportion of the population over sixty-five years of age rose from 4.9 percent in 1950 to 9.0 percent in 1980, and is expected to reach 14 percent by the year 2000, making it comparable with the proportions in Great Britain and Scandinavia (Keizai Kikaku Chōhen 1982). The largest increase has been in the most medically frail sector of the aged, those over seventy-five years of age (D. Maeda 1983).

> National medical costs for the aged rose 600 percent between 1973 and 1982, doubling from 10 percent to 20 percent of total health care costs (JICWELS 1983). U.S. costs roughly quadrupled in the same period (Muse and Sawyer 1982).

> The number of nursing home beds in Japan nearly doubled in the six years between 1977 and 1983, from 55,000 to 97,000 (*Asahi Shimbun* Aug. 29, 1983).

> More than one-fourth of all hospital beds for the acutely ill are occupied by people over the age of seventy (N. Maeda 1983a), and 1.6 percent of those over age sixty-five are in long-term care facilities (Prime Minister's Office 1980), in contrast with America's 5 percent.

In short, this demographic and medical revolution is transforming Japanese life and politics at a dizzying pace. Health laws are enacted and withdrawn; new municipal schemes for cutting the costs of geriatric care are formulated almost daily. Meanwhile, much is left to the unknown legions of families that must care for the disabled elderly. The overall picture, from a distance, is that of a society struggling to find solutions to a sudden, massive problem. One sees an outpouring of popular print and television time devoted to aging and health. One sees a bewildering variety of public and private local organizations doing admirable and sometimes puzzling things to try to improve the lives of the elderly, but with inadequate money and inadequately trained personnel. One also sees, among the healthy elderly, a pervasive anxiety about their own fate as they gradually lose physical and mental vigor.

The brief overview of Japan's geriatric health care system given here cannot begin to document the impact of these demographic changes on individual life. By confining myself to some remarks on the emergence of the "ugly decline" as a social problem and the role of the Japanese government in trying to control it, I hope to provide a useful contrast with the way the problem is being handled in Western societies. Japan provides an interesting point of comparison with the West for two reasons: the first is the speed with which its population is aging; the second is the contrasts it presents to Western cultural views of what is ugly about medical dependency in old age.

National Policy and Health Care Costs

Turning to the problem of government's role, let us first look at recent national policy. Before 1973 national health insurance covered 70 percent of health care costs. The insurance system had its problems, especially for the elderly. Because many of the elderly had no other health insurance, 30 percent of their costs were out-of-pocket. This led to a nationwide call for *rōjin iryō muryōka*, free medical care for the elderly. Insurance reimbursements to physicians are on a "reasonable fee" basis, thereby tempting them to keep their consultations as short as possible (Lock 1980). By 1963 the national government had recognized the growing problem of medical dependency and sought to combat it by detecting and treating diseases of the aged earlier and by establishing a minimum of institutional care for the destitute and chronically ill. In that year the Law for the Welfare of the Aged was passed, ordering municipalities to provide free health screening for those over sixty-five in an effort to promote wellness in this age group and to establish nursing homes for the disabled and homeless elderly. The number of nursing homes nevertheless remains fairly small, for reasons I will discuss later. The results of the health screening policy were disappointing. Less than 20 percent of the elderly participated in the screening in most places (N. Maeda 1983a), partly because many municipalities were short of the funds and personnel required to do the job well. Few of those identified as needing treatment actually showed up in doctors' offices. The general effect was simply to provide free checkups to those who felt sick and would have consulted a doctor anyway. Further attempts to control rates of geriatric illness were made at the national level in 1970 and again in 1974, when blood pressure screening campaigns were announced to combat stroke, the leading cause of disability and death in Japan. These campaigns were also disappointing in their low rates of participation (N. Maeda 1983a).

Under the 1963 law the real difficulty from the government's point of view was not the health of the people but the health of the powerful Liberal Democratic party. In the late 1960s and early 1970s Japan had broken out in local rashes of socialism. Many municipalities (including Tokyo) were offering free medical care for the elderly earlier than the national government. According to Kinoshita (1981), this is largely why, in 1973, the Diet passed an amendment to the welfare act that boosted hospital benefits and made most outpatient services free to those over seventy years of age. In retrospect, this policy seems to have been unsuccessful. The number of the elderly in physicians' waiting rooms immediately doubled and health costs shot up 300 percent in the next four years. Meanwhile, the socialist rash seemed to clear up through the natural process of economic inflation, as local governments floundered in meeting medical service costs.

The worst problem with the 1973 amendment was that although it greatly increased public awareness, it also increased public cost due to the new government support of hospital expenses for the elderly. By 1978 Japan had ninety-five acute care beds per ten thousand persons, about twice the U.S. rate, and a hospital outlay of $41.5 billion per year (Hashimoto 1981; JICWELS 1983); and by 1981 the average hospital stay for acute care of those over age sixty-five was eighty-eight days at a cost of $51 per day (N. Maeda 1983a), as compared with the American average of eleven days at a cost (to Medicare) of about $400 per day (Muse and Sawyer 1982, 26). Apparently the lawmakers' mistake was to think either that medical dependency would be born stoically by the people as before or that it would disappear if enough hospital medicine were available. They failed to see that they were trying to cure a problem that had been created by high-technology medicine—that is, medical dependency—by increasing the supply of high-technology medicine.

By the 1980s Japan was faced with a very threatening trend: the greatly increased use of health resources by the elderly. Unable to see the irony in this application of technical progress, many Japanese blamed the victims, the elderly themselves. Many of the elderly (especially the majority, the healthy ones) also disliked the existing policy, which they saw as somewhat patronizing. In February 1983 a new national policy was adopted to address the hospital cost problem. The Old Age Health Act, as it is called, does five things of interest to us here.

1. It shifts the burden of costs from taxes to the insurance premiums of other, solvent health insurance systems, including society health, mutual aid, and other national programs.
2. It strengthens preventive health care by making low-cost checkups available to those over forty years old.
3. It controls indiscriminate use of services by requiring elderly patients to pay out-of-pocket four hundred yen for the first clinic visit in any given month and three hundred yen for each day of hospitalization.
4. It controls profiteering by hospitals by reimbursing on a diminishing schedule—the longer the stay, the lower the rate.
5. It encourages home care by providing discharge planning, day-care, and home health services.

No one yet knows what the long-term effects of this new plan will be. In the short run it has created a severe demand for nursing home beds, as hospitals scramble to get rid of their chronically ill patients and families are not ready to accept them. In late August 1983 the Ministry of Health and Welfare announced a plan to create a model nursing home in each prefecture, which it was hoped would function to keep standards of care high. But because of a shortage of skilled personnel and space, the job of filling the need for long-term institutional care will be immense.

Health Care Costs at the Local Level

National policy charges so-called primary local authorities with the work of implementing the health insurance programs. These 3,255 local care systems are not uniform. Many communities have access to nursing homes (there are a total of 1,311 in the country); most have medical screening programs; some have home health services. Currently eighty-one local authorities offer day-care programs. The provision of "respite" nursing home beds for periods up to seven days, to relieve families of homebound, bedfast elderly, began in 1978. By 1983 an estimated 28,000 families had participated in this program. As we will see later when we discuss family care, this is one of the most urgently needed services and it is still seriously underdeveloped. I will not describe the variety of local care, but I can give some idea of its flavor by describing two programs that are attracting national attention and, if they succeed, are likely to influence the development of services in other areas. These programs are in Musashino, a suburb of Tokyo, and Sawauchi Mura, a farming village in Iwate prefecture.

Musashino: Resource Management

Musashino is a high-income commuter town of 133,000 people in the Tokyo megalopolitan area. The aged population there is about the national average of 9 percent, or 13,000 people. Three unusual features of the geriatric care system in Musashino have given the city national visibility.

First, the City Medical Association decided against offering the usual mass health screenings, with their usual 20 percent response rate, to the elderly. Instead, in 1971 it began individual screenings in physicians' offices, which resulted in response rates above 50 percent (Yamate 1983). This innovation was made possible by two unusual facts. One, Musashino is relatively rich in physicians, having 2.7 per 1,000 population, over twice the national average (Keizai Keikaku Chōhen 1982, 103). Two, the medical association had the foresight, in 1968, to arrange for use of the business computer of the Fuji Bank for billing services, which made the mass handling of individual health data much easier. This procedure was an important innovation in controlling costs.

A second unusual feature of the city's geriatric care system, begun in April 1981, is the coordination of voluntary and municipal organizations to provide in-home care for the ill elderly. The city welfare office employs five home helpers and four home health nurses, and also refers callers to services provided by the police and fire departments, the Red Cross, and several other volunteer agencies that provide meals and friendly visitors and perform chores. Elders in the community may receive for a reasonable cost at home meals, nursing care, rehabilitation, visitors, help in homemaking and chores, and transportation. Destitute families receive these services free. In addition, the city operates a community center where the elderly may receive day-care and rehabilitation and where beds' are available so that homebound elderly can stay for a few days while their regular caretakers rest.

The third noteworthy feature of the Musashino system is a city-subsidized public corporation that offers health care mortgages. Elderly clients who cannot pay for services but who own property can float mortgages at 5 percent interest and draw upon the money to pay health costs not covered by insurance, including home help, bathing, transportation, meals, rehabilitation, and a variety of other services.

The avowed goal of the screening, home care, and community center programs is to keep health costs down by keeping people out of hospitals. The question is, how well is it working? There are many problems, of which outreach is one. In August of 1983 only 145 people were using the in-home and day-care services in Musashino, a mere 1 percent of the elderly. Since nationwide the rate of serious chronic illness among the elderly seems to be around 12.5 percent and total disability around 4 percent (N. Maeda 1983a), the degree of success appears to be limited. Moreover, as word about these programs has spread to other communities in the Tokyo area, chronically ill people have moved to Musashino in order to make use of them. This circumstance is what might be called one of the costs of living in an information-rich society. It will probably be several years before the financial soundness, or lack of it, of the Musashino plan is well enough established to warrant testing in other localities. Meanwhile, in 1983 Musashino's new mayor seemed determined to reverse what many saw as the socialist policies of the former city government.

Sawauchi Mura: Resource Creation

Sawauchi Mura is a farming town of about five thousand people spread out along twenty-six kilometers of road in the mountains an hour west of Morioka city in the northern prefecture of Iwate. On the whole, it is a nonaffluent, remote, cold place to live. In the 1950s the village had its share of health problems, like most rural villages in the area. Infant mortality rates averaged about fifty per thousand live births, well above the national average, and the population over age sixty-five ran about 5 percent of the total, far below the national average. By 1983 the village had listed its health accomplishments in a published pamphlet titled *The Village of Nature and Health*. Indeed, by the late 1970s the infant mortality rate had fallen to about ten per thousand, and the proportion of elderly had tripled to about 15 percent, one of the highest rates in Iwate prefecture. Even more amazing was that health care expenditures per person in the over-seventy age bracket had dropped to less than half the national average, and just over one-third the average of nearby Morioka city (N. Maeda 1983b).

What had happened? In 1957 an extremely energetic and idealistic man named Fukazawa Masao was elected mayor of Sawauchi. Among his goals was the correction of Sawauchi's health problems. He realized this would take a grass-roots effort, since outside money would be hard to come by. In 1958 he established a pension for villagers over seventy years of age. Two years later he established a policy, financed by local taxes, of making supplementary payments to national health insurance claims for children and old people. This policy made their health care essentially free, constituting a comprehensive, prepaid medical plan for the high-risk members of the village (N. Maeda 1983b). Soon afterward other municipalities also adopted this policy of *rōjin iryō muryōka*.

Fukazawa died in 1965, only seven years after taking office; but he had touched off a process that has continued to gain momentum. In 1983, under a new mayor, Sawauchi was receiving daily out-of-town health professionals, planners, and scholars seeking a better understanding of what the village had achieved. At that time Sawauchi had its own health center with forty-six beds and a daily outpatient load of 178. Health screening of the elderly was aggressive. All village residents were periodically scheduled for two days of combined testing and health education at the clinic, in groups of six to eight. Participation in these screenings was running about 60 percent for males and higher for women. Mass screenings for high blood pressure and cancer, I was told, were reaching 80 to 90 percent of the elderly (although I noticed that only about half the eligible participants showed up for a screening at which I was present). All village residents were being encouraged to drop in to the health center for an interview with a nurse whenever they liked, whether seriously ill or not, and staff members were trained to make them feel comfortable. Public health nurses were making calls on bedfast patients at home, at the same time collecting health information on others in the household and disseminating health data. Several of the twelve *buraku* (residential subdivisions) of the village had volunteer visitor groups to check on the sick and report to the health center. Clinic nurses made routine stops at the homes of patients on their way home from work to drop off medicine and collect current health information. As of 1983, there were several self-help groups (for example, for stroke patients, diabetics, and for families of psychiatric patients). In addition to lay social workers *(minsei-iin)*, each *buraku* had a team of lay health workers *(hoken-iin)*, elected by the residents. The role of the *hoken-iin* includes getting people to come to the health screenings, reporting health hazards in their neighborhood, and counseling residents on the use of the village health system.

As one may infer from the energy that Sawauchi expends on health care, its leaders seem to have succeeded in making health a subject of everyday thought for most of the villagers. They have become aware of their own previously unexamined attitudes and behavior with respect to health and illness; and they have likewise become aware of their neighbors' attitudes. In this atmosphere, self-ignorance, self-neglect, and self-abuse become visible forms of deviance and are subject to much the same social pressures that might control laziness, wife beating, and other socially undesirable tendencies. The smallness, homogeneity, stability, and traditionalism of the village have been turned into resources for the control of illness and the minimizing of health care costs. There are echoes here of the kind of ideological groupthink that has been described in some rural religious "utopias" (Plath 1966, 1969), to be sure, but there also are major differences. One difference is that Sawauchi is not addressing an eccentrically personal spiritual vision, but a problem that is increasingly front-page news, not only in Japan but throughout the world. As a result, one gets the feeling that the achievement of concrete goals takes precedence over pious attitudes or conformity for its own sake, although the latter are also important at times.

Many aspects of Sawauchi's system are being studied and adopted by other communities in Japan, but it is difficult to predict how they will fare elsewhere. Many Sawauchi residents seem to identify themselves closely with their community and with the goals set by its now semilegendary leader, Fukazawa. Their loyalty to their health care system is evident.[1]

Stress in Families

We now turn from the measured, tabulated, and published costs of geriatric care to the largely unmeasureable and invisible costs: stress in families of the chronically and terminally ill. There can be no doubt about the importance of assessing these costs. The very difficulty of measuring them results in the false images of robust social justice and enviable wealth that are invoked by statistics on increasing longevity.

To begin with, there is the question of numbers. How many chronically ill or bedfast elderly are cared for at home? In contrast with European countries and the United States, it is still the expectation of Japanese policymakers and the public that the dependent elderly will be cared for at home by their families. Based on the number of those diagnosed chronically ill with typical diseases of the elderly and the number of elderly living with their families (JICWELS 1983; Keizai Kikaku Chōhen 1982; N. Maeda 1983a), I estimate there are about 1.3 million cases of geriatric chronic illness represented among families with an elderly member. About 438,000 of these elderly are bedfast, and of the bedfast, 307,000 live with their families (D. Maeda 1983). Seventy-four percent of the bedfast have been incapacitated for more than six months (Soda and Miura 1982).

When co-residence with the family is impossible, a variety of institutions is available for the dependent elderly that correspond roughly to our institutions—residential, intermediate, and skilled nursing facilities. These are subsidized by the government under the 1963 Welfare of the Elderly Law. Aside from the relatively small number of these institutions, there is a major difference between Japan and the West in the way they are used. In the West, we have a "pull" model of institutionalization: the patient needs a certain kind of care, and the services of the institution are sought to fill these needs. In Japan, by contrast, a "push" model is more usual: the family cannot care for the patient, usually for economic or logistic reasons, so he or she must go somewhere. This difference is illustrated by the key role of the physician in the decision to institutionalize in the West, and, in this matter, his relative unimportance in Japan, where referral and admission to long-term care is often arranged by social workers without the participation of a physician. The assumption seems to be that for anything short of acute hospital care, family care is ipso facto best, unless the family is physically or economically unable to give care at all. This view, plus the fact that the rate of long-term institutionalization in Japan is 1.6 percent of those over sixty-five (versus 5 percent in the United States), reveals a set of Japanese norms and social conditions that say, "Thou shalt care for thy dependent elderly relatives."

Self-help groups are available in most major metropolitan areas for most serious chronic illnesses. Family members of demented elderly, for example, have a national association with twenty-one branches and about a thousand members, the great majority of whom are in the Tokyo, Kyoto, and Osaka areas. Members of this association hold monthly meetings, during which they hear lectures on matters of care of the aged and offer moral support to one another. The association is similar to the Alzheimer's Disease and Related Disorders Association (ADRDA) in the United States, with two major predictable differences: first, the Japanese association includes families of those with theoretically treatable dementias; and second, it seems to pay little attention to diagnosis or rehabilitation. The greater availability of self-help groups in the urban area may reflect the relative need for volunteer help in those areas where work takes family members away from the home more often. One study (Otani et al. 1983) found that rural families are better able to support the elderly ill at home and that, unexpectedly, community services for the bedfast elderly are more available in some rural areas.

Who are the caretakers of the dependent elderly? Various studies (Nakajima, Saito, and Tsukihashi 1982; Shimizu 1982; D. Maeda 1983) show that the largest category of caretakers for elderly men is their wives, and for women, it is daughters-in-law. Fewer than 10 percent of caretakers are men. A fourth of all caretakers are over the age of sixty (D. Maeda 1983). In the study conducted by Nakajima, Saito, and Tsukihashi, 63 percent were over age fifty.

While it is impossible to make firm generalizations on the degree of stress suffered by families of the elderly ill, in a study reported by D. Maeda (1983), well over half the families caring for the elderly with a wide range of disabilities characterized their situation as "very difficult." Nakajima, Saito, and Tsukihashi's (1982) subjects were members of a self-help society dealing with a relatively high-stress illness (dementia), and it is probably safe to assume that their stress level is higher than average. Ninety-two percent of the caretakers said they felt some distress in their roles; 54 percent rated their stress as acute; and 50 percent said caretaking was a round-the-clock job. Feelings of caretakers toward their role are of special interest. In the Nakajima, Saito, and Tsukihashi study, 77 percent of the caretakers said they wanted to continue; but of these, about a fifth said they did not see how they could. Another 22 percent of the sample did not want to continue their role but saw no way out of it. The more time-consuming the caretaking, the less inclined people were to want to quit. The older the caretakers were, the less likely they were to feel their service was a sacrifice. On the whole, the picture one gets from these data is supported by conversations with family members of ill elderly persons. The circumstances do not seem very different from those in the United States. Most caretakers are willing to take on the responsibilities, but they are often frustrated by conflicting demands such as those of child rearing and occupational work and by the lack of helpful resources outside the family. Older people and those with fewer conflicting demands seem most committed to the caretaker role.

The use of, and desire for, outside help is another measure of the stress associated with the caretaker role. Nakajima, Saito, and Tsukihashi (1982) found a considerable unfilled need in this respect, as did Shimizu (1982) and Otani and his colleagues (1983). For example, only 3 percent of the Nakajima, Saito, and Tsukihashi sample had access to respite care, while 33.6 percent felt a need for it. Only 1.6 percent had access to daycare, while 20 percent wanted this service. The magnitude of this problem can be appreciated, however, only when the level of tolerance for stress is understood. D. Maeda's study (1983, 582) found that "less than half of the families who were judged as needing home help service stated that they wanted to use that service." The most frequently used service, telephone consultation, was used by only 13 percent of the Nakajima, Saito, and Tsukihashi sample. In another study, Nakajima (personal communication 1983) found that the most frequent problem of people calling for help with a demented patient was the need for a diagnosis of the problem. In fact, 43 percent of 145 callers had been unable to get any diagnosis at all. (An interesting footnote to this study was that many calls came from patients' daughters, who were not the primary caretakers, probably because daughters are often key decision makers for the elderly parents even when they do not live in the same household.)

The Japanese health care system appears to leave a great deal of responsibility for care to the family. This care is often extremely onerous, but most caretakers accept it as their role, either out of personal conviction or as a result of community pressure. What most family caretakers seem to want first is the comfort and well-being of the parent; after that, they would like knowledge about the likely course of the illness, followed by the desire for occasional relief from the strain of caretaking, and finally, rehabilitative treatment for the parent. The development of outside services for the caretaker families lags well behind provisions for their need for information and respite. Rehabilitative treatment programs are even farther off.

Culture and the "Ugly Decline"

Up to this point I have been describing the demographic and economic problem of a medically created geriatric population and recent attempts of Japanese society to deal with that problem through the instrument of public policy. But the problem, of course, is not merely a demographic and economic one. We are talking about the suffering of those who are ill and the injustice of the fact that some of them are well cared for by family and have ready access to professional help while others do not. The ideas of "suffering" and "injustice" are in part culturally defined. Finding acceptable solutions to such problems means finding solutions that make sense given the cultural norms that pertain to the comfort, dignity, and civil rights of the aged. Clearly, just enabling more people to live longer under any circumstances is not an acceptable use of medical technology in Japan or any other society. The "ugly decline" is ugly because it violates cultural norms, and ugliness on such a large scale is not acceptable. The question to which I now turn is what is ugly about the lives of the medically dependent aged from the Japanese point of view, and how does this point of view affect policy regarding geriatric health care?

A major difference between Japanese and Western models of geriatric care is that hospitalized elderly in Japan remain in hospital much longer than those in the West, and there are fewer facilities for the care or rehabilitation of the chronically ill elderly. In 1977 a grand total of 7,251 old people were getting any kind of rehabilitation, less than 3 percent of the total number of bedfast elderly (Prime Minister's Office 1980, 194). Is there anything cultural about these facts, aside from the obvious conclusion that the Japanese still allocate to the family many responsibilities we Westerners have come to see as public?

Let us first look at some economic conditions and historical facts. The long hospital stays and the lack of long-term care beds are obviously related. Until nursing homes are built, severely and chronically ill people have to live somewhere in a society that keeps them alive artificially. Since World War II the cost of land and construction in Japan has been extremely high, pushing upward the cost of building nursing homes. This condition does not explain much, however, because care in nursing homes is still cheaper than in hospitals, even when current building costs are figured in. There is also the problem of politics. The method of reimbursing nursing homes for patient care cost is the subject of debate between the Liberal Democrats (who want to charge families on a sliding scale) and the opposition parties, who want the services to be covered by welfare. This debate tends to delay the development of the industry. Another political problem, mentioned in Long's chapter in this volume, is the relatively great power of the Japan Medical Association and the unwillingness of physicians to transfer authority to other helping professions. Nursing home care, home care, and day-care will only work in societies where there is a good supply of well-trained nurses and health paraprofessionals, and this supply can only develop where the work of these professionals is encouraged and legitimized by those in power.

Historical associations fuel the political debate and lend an unfortunate symbolism to nursing homes. There is a historical connection between modern nursing homes and their predecessor institutions, the *yōrō in,* which were mainly poor houses not medical facilities. The opposition parties argue that no one should have to pay to enter a poor house. Many people associate nursing homes with the shame of poverty, although the skilled nursing facilities are open to middle-class families. Again, this fact doesn't explain why many middle-class people do place their parents in nursing homes or why Japan's nursing homes offer rehabilitation to only 4.4 percent of their patients (Prime Minister's Office 1980, 194).

Still another historical factor is the double structure of the hospital industry. About a sixth of Japan's acute care beds are in small private clinics with fewer than twenty beds each (JICWELS 1983). Here, the hospitalizing physician stands to gain personally by keeping the beds filled, much like the physician-owners of many U.S. proprietary nursing homes. But even if stays in these hospitals are unusually long (no precise data on this matter are available), one-sixth is not a large proportion, implying that economic conditions of the small private clinics cannot be the only influencing factor. The government's preferred explanation for long stays is that people overuse hospitals because they are free. This would be convincing only if many people preferred hospitalization to other living arrangements, which I do not think is the case.

The lack of rehabilitation services might be explained simply by a lack of financial incentives to develop them. As long as the medical professionals are making money, perhaps they do not perceive a problem in this area. However, long hospital stays definitely are a problem for the government, the taxpayers, and the disabled elderly themselves. Other so-called aging societies like England, Sweden, and Holland have made great strides in rehabilitation medicine due largely to economic incentives. If the incentive argument is to be convincing, we must be able to see evidence that either the medical establishment is disproportionately powerful in Japan or that there are cultural barriers to thinking about rehabilitation at the policy level.

Let us turn, then, to the Japanese cultural factors that give low priority to rehabilitation. These factors must be sought systematically in the way people treat old age, chronic illness, and health care. Let me cite some pertinent facts and observations.

1. There are admirable transportation aids and rehabilitation centers for the ambulatory and the independently living impaired. They are not a "neglected" minority.
2. On the geriatric care circuit, one hears over and over a word that has almost disappeared in the West—the word "bedridden" *(netakiri)*—used as though it were a permanent condition.
3. One often sees the stroke patient, the most frequent example of *netakiri,* being lovingly fed, massaged, and talked to, but wasting away in the hospital or in the sickroom bed at home.
4. At the showing of a film on dementia, one viewer, herself the wife of a stroke patient, said, "I didn't like the way the nurse was pushing the old lady to 'do this,' and 'do that.' If they don't naturally want to be healthy again, pushing them won't change things."
5. When one asks members of the rural old folks' club what their biggest worry is, someone says, "That we should become *netakiri,"* and others nod.
6. The splendid new residential homes for the aged that are sprouting up everywhere lack facilities for rehabilitation, or even plans for adding them. The advertisements for one planned facility in Kobe show a schedule of pro-rated refunds if the buyer gets chronically sick during the first ten years of residence. It is evidently expected that chronic illness means, naturally, that he would have to leave. The builders of these facilities have studied the Danish and British and Dutch models, but they have rejected the concept of a continuum-of-care.

Much has been written about Japanese norms for expressing and gratifying dependence needs (Caudill 1962; Doi 1973; Lebra 1976; Reynolds 1976). I might summarize these writings by saying that there are several well-developed role sets in the culture that encourage passive helplessness by one partner and active nurturing by the other, and that sickness and caretaking are one such role set. The caretaker is actively solicitous of the patient's emotional as well as physical needs. This circumstance is somewhat different from the American/Northwest European tradition, wherein the patient feels a strong aversion to his own passivity and presumably feels better emotionally through the simple process of becoming more active and mobile (Strauss 1975; Zborowski 1969).

This Japanese role set is expressed also in Japanese and other East Asian forms of treatment. Illness is felt to be a problem of imbalance between the individual and his environment, an abnormality in the flow of energy (Caudill 1976). In contrast with the aggressive methods of Western medicine, where treatment often adds considerably to the patient's discomfort, Eastern methods aim more at adjusting the relationship between the patient and his environment and are more likely to be gentle and nonintrusive. If possible, they should even be pleasant, and they are likely to involve the diligent work of nurturant healing figures over long periods. This is true of herbalism and many forms of acupuncture, moxibustion, massage, and the Japanese psychotherapies (Lock 1980; Reynolds 1980). The best parallel in Western medicine is analytically based psychotherapy, the one form of treatment where the fostering of dependence is felt to be an important, if temporary, part of the cure.

Disability, as Sigerist (1932) pointed out, is an anomaly in Western civilization because the patient cannot get well and thereby violates the patient-healer role set. By contrast, rehabilitation of the bedfast is an anomaly in Japanese culture because it often requires the caretaker to violate the emotional terms of the role set. Rehabilitation requires the imposition of discomfort on the patient, and on some extent the patient's rejection of nurturing by the caregiver. Moreover, this anomaly is especially marked in cases where the caregiver and the patient are members of the same family. The professional caregiver role more often includes a mandate to impose discomfort when scientific knowledge indicates that a therapeutic result cannot otherwise be achieved.

This cultural promotion of dependency applies to people of all ages. It becomes a problem in the case of the aged because their health problems tend to be multiple and their capacity to recover is impaired. They take longer to recover, and they tend to recover less function than young people. To take a simple example, compare a 30-year-old and a 75-year-old who have fallen and broken a leg. (Falls are a leading cause of hospitalization in people over age sixty-five.) The young person will probably recover near-total functioning in a few weeks with little or no rehabilitation therapy. The old person, however, may never recover 100 percent of functioning because of poor healing. She is also likely to have balance problems due to loss of central nervous system function, and/or arthritis, and/or vision impairment, and/or drug-related disorientation. Her recovery is likely to take practice, muscle development, and training in the use of a walker or cane. She may not be able to return to her former home without modification of steps and walkways and appliances, and in her impaired condition she is likely to fear walking alone. Overcoming all these barriers to independence will require courage and determination on the patient's part. She is likely to lapse into depression, which, in turn, must be treated.

In a culture like that of the United States or England, where full autonomy is considered a right and an obligation that is only temporarily affected by illness, motivation to carry out this stressful process will be high for both the therapist and the patient. In a culture lacking this view of human relations, motivation may not always be up to the task.

At first glance this interpretation seems to conflict with other evidence that suggests that helpless dependency is an unpleasant experience for the aged and for their caretakers alike. Plath (1972), for example, describes the *"pokkuri jinja,"* shrines where old people go to pray for a speedy death. And there is the well-known *"Obaasute-yama"* (*"Granny-flinging Mountain"*) legend, in which a family takes a healthy but superannuated grandmother to a lonely mountain crag and abandons her. I do not think these bits of tradition pose a problem for the interpretation I am suggesting. For one thing, as Plath (1972) has noted, such traditions speak of the deep ambivalence with which aging and the aged are regarded in any society. Customs and other norms often make people miserable, and they are often used to justify antisocial impulses as well. Passivity or nurturing can be just as unpleasant in a passivity-fostering culture as in a passivity-fearing one when one is not in the mood to be passive or nurturant. Both old people and their children fear illness more in a culture like that of Japan, which does not customarily offer them the choice of striving for independence or of not doing so.

In short, old people tend to stay in Japanese hospitals for a long time partly because very little effort is made to get them up and out. This lack of effort stems partly from the fact that rehabilitation conflicts with the caretaker's mandate to give emotional succor and the patient's mandate to passively receive it. The strength of these cultural prescriptions in a society still as homogenous and as public as Japan's is gives a characteristic expression to the fears surrounding the chronic illness of old age. Understanding norms that govern the relationships of parent and child, caretaker and patient, helps us to explain why the Japanese search for solutions to the technologically created "ugly decline" has taken the path I have described. Culturally, ugliness in this case is defined not as Western culture defines it, namely, the loss of control over one's own fate; rather, what is ugly is the prolonged activation of obligatory roles wherein the caretaker must give succor in heroic measure and the patient must passively receive it.

Future Prospects

Gerontologist Daisaku Maeda concludes a recent article on care of the elderly with a concise statement of the outlook for the near future in Japan.

> The family is, and will continue to be, the most important source of support for the elderly in Japan. In the future, however, the relative importance of family support of the elderly will inevitably decrease because (1) the proportion and real number of frail and impaired older people who are no longer independent in their daily living will greatly increase and (2) the capability of families to care for older parents will decrease due to industrialization and urbanization. Therefore, various social services for the frail and impaired elderly and support services for the families who care for them will undoubtedly have to be expanded. (D. Maeda 1983, 583)

This obviously implies a further turn of the screw, escalating public responsibility and public cost in an effort to compensate for the unwanted effects of technological progress. We might deplore this if there were any alternative in sight, but there is not; it is fundamental to the process of economic development in which all advanced nations now find themselves. But we can ask what negative effects this coming escalation is likely to have on the quality of life. Will it further disfigure the image of old age and death, and if so, how? There are likely to be both gains and losses. On the negative side, the lives of many severely ill and helpless old people will be prolonged by the creation of professional services to care for them. This is the very situation that wedded the image of old age to the spectre of medical dependency in the first place. It is unlikely that the new nursing homes and family support programs will include vigorous attempts to rehabilitate the chronically ill, for reasons I have discussed. Such attempts, if undertaken, may shorten the period of

helplessness and thereby improve the quality of late life. A second negative effect of the coming changes is a likely reduction in the quality of life
for many of the growing population of elderly who will spend months or
years in nursing homes. Even the best nursing home can scarcely offer
the variety and flexibility of care or the familiar and personally meaningful surroundings of the many private homes from which its patients have
ultimately come, and to which most of them long to return.

On the positive side, much can be said as well. Most important, services to families will allow more ill elderly to remain in familiar surroundings and at the same time reduce the suffering of many family
caretakers. Second, the development of nursing homes now, with our
current medical, psychological, and social knowledge of chronic illness,
offers hope that patients will receive more humane and better-informed
care than has been offered up to now in geriatric hospitals. Many current
hospital wards for the elderly have grown out of urgent necessity, without
adequate planning. Yet another possible benefit of the future is that it
will require the development of new and better approaches to the care of
the chronically ill. Some European countries, notably Great Britain, the
Netherlands, and Sweden, are developing a team approach to geriatric
care. In this approach physicians share responsibility with other experts
whose job is to minimize medical dependency—physical and occupational therapists, nutritionists, nurses, and social workers. This appears
to be an economical and humane alternative to high-technology, hospital-based medicine. If the team approach is used properly, it can promote independence and free choice among the elderly by keeping them
out of institutions and off drugs and by helping them and their families
to cope with their disabilities.

The basic conditions of industrial civilization have added permanently
to the human life-cycle a prolonged period of decline. Too often that
decline is "ugly" because we have been too busy postponing death to
confront the quality of life that results from our efforts. So far, Japan is
no exception.

Notes

Data for this report were collected chiefly during the month of August, 1983, in
Japan. Whatever worthwhile results that month produced I owe to the extraordi-
nary kindness and impressive knowledge of Professor Maeda Nobuo, Head, Sec-
tion of Social Security, Institute of Public Health, Tokyo; to Dr. Saito Kazuko,
Head, Section on Aging, National Institute of Mental Health, Ichikawa; and to
Kinoshita Yasuhito, who recently completed his Ph.D. in Human Development

and Aging, UCSF, and to the dozens of health care workers, city officials, and elderly patients they introduced me to.
  1. The following example shows the loyalty of villagers to the system. Central to the operation of the care system of the village is the fact that the staff members of the health center know all the patients personally. This personal knowledge assures continuity and coordination of services that (as other local systems show) would otherwise become very fragmented. Building up personal knowledge of the clients, in turn, requires very low rates of turnover among health center staff members. The two nurses presently working in the ambulatory care center both grew up in Sawauchi, and both have worked there since they left nursing school. When I asked the director of operations of the center the secret of such loyalty, he said proudly, "The philosophy established by Mr. Fukazawa twenty-six years ago is still almost unchanged. It has continued to develop and spread."

References

Caudill, W. 1962. Patterns of emotion in modern Japan. In *Japanese culture,* ed. R. J. Smith and R. K. Beardsley. Chicago: Aldine.
————. 1976. The cultural and interpersonal context of everyday health and illness in Japan. In *Asian medical systems,* ed. C. Leslie. Berkeley and Los Angeles: Univ. of California Press.
Doi, T. 1973. *The anatomy of dependence.* Tokyo: Kodansha.
Hashimoto, M. 1981. National health administration in Japan. *Bulletin of the Institute of Public Health* 30 (1): 1–26.
Japan International Corporation of Welfare Services (JICWELS). 1983. *Trends and policies of health services in Japan.* Tokyo: JICWELS.
Kamata, K., et al. 1983. Problems in the process of the bedridden elderly in the community. *Shakai Rōnengaku* 17:97–107.
Keizai Kikaku Chōhen. 1982. *Kokumin seikatsu hakusho* (White paper on national life). Tokyo: Ōkurasho Printing Office.
Kinoshita, Y. 1981. Now you see it, now you don't. Paper presented at the thirty-fourth annual meeting of the Gerontological Society of America, Nov. 8–12, Toronto, Canada.
Lebra, T. 1976. *Japanese patterns of behavior.* Honolulu: Univ. of Hawaii Press.
Lock, M. 1980. *East Asian medicine in urban Japan.* Berkeley and Los Angeles: Univ. of California Press.
Maeda, D. 1983. Family care in Japan. *The Gerontologist* 23 (6): 579–583.
Maeda, N. 1983a. Health schemes for the aged in Japan. Scientific Session Papers, Ninth Joint Tokyo/New York Medical Congress, Tokyo.
————. 1983b. *Medical care in Sawauchi Mura, Iwate prefecture.* Tokyo: Nihon Hyōron.

Muse, D., and D. Sawyer. 1982. *Health care financing, program statistics.* Washington D.C.: Dept. of Health and Human Services.

Nakajima, K., K. Saito, and Y. Tsukihashi. 1982. Boke rōjin to sono kazoku no jittai (Actual conditions of the demented elderly and their families). *Hokenfu Zasshi* 38 (12): 10–47.

Okura, T. 1983. Implementing communal medical care for the elderly. Scientific Session Papers, Ninth Joint Tokyo/New York Medical Congress, Tokyo.

Otani, M., et al. 1983. A case study on family care of the aged with diseases. *Shakai Rōnengaku* 17:83–90.

Plath, D. 1966. The fate of Utopia. *American Anthropologist* 68 (5): 1152–1162.

———. 1969. Modernization and its discontents—Japan's little utopias. *Journal of Asian and African Studies* 4 (1): 1–17.

———. 1972. Japan, the after years. In *Aging and modernization,* ed. D. O. Cowgill and L. D. Holmes. New York: Appleton-Century-Crofts.

———. 1973. Cares of career, and careers of caretaking. *Journal of Nervous and Mental Diseases* 157 (5): 346–357.

———. 1980. *Long engagements.* Stanford: Stanford Univ. Press.

———. 1983. Ecstasy years—old age in Japan. In *Growing old in different societies,* ed. J. Sokolovsky. Belmont, Calif.: Wadsworth.

Prime Minister's Office. 1980. *Koreisha mondai no genjō* (The present state of the problems of the elderly). Sōrifu, Tokyo: Okura-sho.

Reynolds, D. 1976. *Morita psychotherapy.* Berkeley and Los Angeles: Univ. of California Press.

———. 1980. *The quiet therapies.* Honolulu: Univ. of Hawaii Press.

Shimizu, Y. 1982. Analysis of factors influencing need expression for home-help services among families caring for the impaired elderly. *Shakai Rōnengaku* 16:10–19.

Sigerist, H. 1932. *Man and medicine.* New York: Norton.

Soda, N., and B. Miura. 1982. *Zuzetsu rōjin hakushō* (Illustrated white paper on aging). Tokyo: Sekibusha.

Sparks, D. E. 1973. Retirement and the relocation of older workers. *Area Development in Japan* 7:24–33.

———. 1975. The still rebirth. *Journal of Asian and African Studies* 10 (1–2): 64–74.

Steslicke, W. E. 1984. Medical care for Japan's aging population. *Pacific Affairs* 57:45–52.

Strauss, A. 1975. *Chronic illness and the quality of life.* St. Louis: C. V. Mosby.

Yamate, S. 1983. Medical examination system for the elderly. Scientific Session Papers, Ninth Joint Tokyo/New York Medical Congress, Tokyo.

Zborowski, M. 1969. *People in pain.* San Francisco: Jossey-Bass.

Japanese Models of Psychotherapy

David K. Reynolds

Historical Background

Although modern psychotherapeutic forms are relatively recent contributions to dealing with human suffering in Japan, their roots extend deeply into Japan's history. A brief examination of the history of Japanese psychotherapeutic practices may contribute to our understanding of the conceptual framework that the therapist and layperson bring to the therapeutic encounter.

Prehistoric evidence indicates that trepanation was practiced during the Neolithic period, perhaps as treatment for mental disturbance. Herbs, poultices, hot baths, cold baths, steam baths, moxibustion (the burning of moxa powder on energy points of the skin), pine needle fumigation, fasting, acupuncture, acupressure, bloodletting, and ingestion of the blood of poisonous snakes were used psychotherapeutically from earliest recorded times. Diet and rest were offered at specialized Buddhist temples.

Shamanism has been practiced in Japan since prehistoric times (Sasaki 1969). By the early twentieth century, common treatments for mental illness included hypnosis, autohypnosis, breathing exercises, prayer, suggestion, bed rest, physical exercises, life-style training, work therapy, travel, massage, and various religious exercises. Psychoanalysis was introduced around 1920 but has never become popular as a mode of treatment.

German-Austrian medicine dominated Japanese psychiatry during the late nineteenth and early twentieth centuries (Bowers 1965). The emphasis on a narrow diagnosis and biological approaches to psychotherapy still predominates in the medical universities today, although interest in mentalistic treatment forms has increased since the introduction and influence of American medicine in the early 1950s. Electroconvulsive treatment and insulin shock therapy were quite commonly practiced until the 1970s, when concerns with patients' rights initiated a reevaluation of their appropriateness. Tranquilizers, antidepressants, and lithium are commonly prescribed; sophistication in psychopharmacology is at least on the level of that in the United States.

Physical facilities for the treatment of the mentally disturbed remained primitive well into the twentieth century. The Law of Confinement and Protection of the Mentally Ill, enacted in 1900, provided for the construction and maintenance of private cells for the mentally ill in their family homes. In 1919 the numbers of persons in mental hospitals and in private dwellings were nearly equal, and as late as 1950, 2,671 people were confined in cells in their homes (Kumasaka and Yoshioka 1968). Since 1950, however, a new law has required hospitalization rather than home confinement. Special instructional facilities for the developmentally disabled have been in operation since 1956. Community psychiatry, residential care facilities, day-care centers, and halfway houses have never found favor in Japan.

In 1975 there were 276,159 beds in over a thousand mental hospitals in Japan, nearly one-quarter of the total hospital beds in that country (see Ikegami 1980 for a full discussion of the growth of inpatient psychiatric facilities in Japan). Today the great majority of psychiatric inpatients are treated in private psychiatric hospitals of less than three hundred beds. Each hospital generally has some connection with a university medical school that is a major source of its referrals for admission.

Current Status

In order to discover Japanese therapists' views of the current status of Japanese psychotherapy, I prepared a set of open-ended questions regarding the most influential therapists and the most influential therapies in Japan today and outstanding changes in Japanese psychotherapy during the past five to ten years. Ten interviews with knowledgeable therapists from a number of universities yielded responses that were much the same, if colored somewhat by my informants' university and professional affiliations.

In response to a broad question regarding influential persons, my informants frequently asked whether I was interested in those who wield power in therapeutic circles, conduct research, and contribute theory, or those who actually practice psychotherapy and have written about their practice. For the most part the names given to me were persons who have done both. In terms of therapeutic preference, most of those mentioned have a psychoanalytic background. Of the nine therapists most frequently named, three are Freudians, one is a Jungian, and each of the remaining five specializes in another mode or specialty area of therapy: Nishizono (Kyushu University), Doi (recently retired from the Japanese National Institute of Mental Health), and Okonogi (Keio University) are Freudians; Kawai (Kyoto University) is a Jungian; other names included Kora (Morita therapy), Yoshimoto (Naikan therapy), Nakai (schizophrenia therapy), Kasahara (adolescent therapy), and Kato (cross-cultural therapy).

As for influential therapies, the respondents distinguished between those favored by psychiatrists and those favored by others. Psychoanalytic styles of therapy are in favor among psychiatrists, particularly Japanese versions of Freudian therapy emphasizing psychodynamically oriented counseling. Among psychologists, social workers, and counselors, there is more interest in Jungian psychoanalysis, nondirective Rogerian therapy, autogenic training, behavior therapy, biofeedback, hypnosis, transactional analysis, group therapies, art therapies, Morita therapy, and Naikan. Some psychiatrists also use these modes of therapy in an eclectic way. It is noteworthy that no physician considered psychopharmacology to be a form of psychotherapy, yet dispensing medication is the primary medical response to mental disorder in Japan, as it is in the United States.

An examination of the stock list of the major distributor of medical books in English gives an idea of the topics and therapies of interest to psychiatrists in Japan. Neurology and neuropsychiatry merit a whole section in the catalog. Biological, biochemical, and somatopsychic approaches to psychiatry are next in frequency. Then come general works on psychiatry and volumes devoted to specific disorders, of which schizophrenia, depression, epilepsy, and sleep disorders are particularly noticeable. Books focused on psychopharmacology follow in frequency. Other specific psychotherapeutic approaches are represented by a few books each on hypnosis, psychoanalysis, electroconvulsive therapy, family therapy, and perhaps ten volumes on behavior therapy. Books about child psychiatry, developmental disorders, and addictions (including alcoholism) are about equally represented with less than ten volumes each. There are a few books each on sociopathy, social aspects of mental health, and aging. I suspect that the order of frequency of topics on this list would not appreciably differ from that in most psychiatry departments in the United States. The emphasis is clearly on biological (including neurological) and chemical approaches to the understanding and treatment of mental disorder in contrast to verbal approaches.

Informants also showed remarkable consistency in their evaluations of developments in Japanese psychotherapy during the past five to ten years. Many pointed to the variety of therapies practiced in Japan today, including versions of many Western forms of psychotherapy. Among these methods in current use are psychoanalysis, short-term therapy, crisis intervention approaches, transactional analysis, group therapy, family therapy, couples counseling, gestalt therapy, encounter groups, logotherapy, sensitivity training, and behavior therapy (Doi 1978). Most of these therapies have undergone modification to make them more suitable to Japanese patients and therapists. For example, transactional analysis in Japan finds more positive value in the "parent" aspect of the self than does Western transactional analysis (Ikemi and Sugita 1975). And Japanese encounter groups and sensitivity training programs tend to be "softer" and more supportive in orientation than their Western counterparts. As experience with a variety of therapies has lengthened, so too has a more critical understanding of their application. Fifteen years ago the psychotherapy journals carried introductory articles on these therapies; now they include more specialized reports on the effectiveness and subproblems of these approaches.

Another trend that can be observed is the rapid entry of psychologists and other professionals and nonprofessionals into this field, once completely dominated by psychiatrists. The new therapists tend to be younger and to be attached to public agencies associated with the Ministries of Health and Welfare, Education, and Justice. They work in schools and institutions for the handicapped and in some clinics, usually in nonpermanent positions. However, because psychiatrists alone among psychotherapists can be reimbursed through health insurance, private practice by therapists other than psychiatrists is rare. It may be said that both psychologists and caseworkers in social welfare have broadened the definitions of their capabilities over the past fifteen years from roles as specialists in psychological testing and social welfare, respectively, into the field of individual and group therapy.

In general, there has been a surge of interest in the possibilities of verbal psychotherapy for clients and practitioners. Interest in the therapeutic applications of art (drawing, modeling, dance, painting, calligraphy, etc.) is matched by a new look at psychoanalysis, particularly Jungian analysis, and, as these have attracted attention in the West, a serious reconsideration of indigenous Japanese therapies. Unfortunately, the interest is not matched by facilities for supervised training. There are very few adequately trained therapists in Japan, whether physicians or those in other fields, and no licensing is required to practice therapy. Beyond some very minimal level, skills are developed as the therapist accumulates experience on the job. Most of my informants mentioned this problem as a key concern for the future of psychotherapy in Japan.

The Japanese Clinical Psychological Association (Nihon Shinri Rinshō Gakkai) was refounded in 1982 following its breakup in 1969 due to internal political disputes. Twelve hundred persons attended the first meeting in October 1982. With the spread of psychologists into a domain once considered to be the exclusive realm of psychiatry, some sort of power struggle might be expected. No clash has yet occurred, probably because of the strong position of physicians in Japan, but the conflict that is currently occurring in the United States must inevitably be repeated in Japan on some level.

Changing Symptom Patterns

Psychotherapies must adapt to fit the changing form of symptoms and complaints of patients. In Japan over the past forty years, neurotic complaints regarding fear of blushing have decreased and phobias concerning eye contact have increased (Maruyama et al. 1982). A number of therapists remarked on the recent increase in neurotic depression—not a true clinical depression but a sort of neurotic discomfort with depressive affect. What seems to have fostered these changes?

Some therapists believe that as shyness has decreased among young people the fear of blushing has become less of a concern for them. One therapist pointed out that fifteen or twenty years ago it was not uncommon to see high school baseball players tremble when they took part in televised ball games. These days they appear more relaxed. Difficulty relating to others remains, however, and some observers believe that the resultant self-consciousness has found more common expression in eye contact phobia. I suspect that this interpretation ignores an important element of self-concealment. The Japanese people are careful about what they reveal to others concerning their thoughts and feelings. Except under special circumstances (for example, when drinking) it is regarded as both thoughtless and potentially troublesome to expose one's inner concerns and emotions (particularly those that might appear to be unsympathetic or otherwise unacceptable). Pervasive fads such as wearing clothing and carrying purses or briefcases of the same styles and discussing the same newspaper and magazine articles may be seen as acceptable ways of concealing fear of personal deficiency through overt uniformity. Blushing reveals to others one's inner turmoil, and so some Japanese make extreme efforts to control it. My guess is that the variety of situations that provoke blushing has decreased as urban Japanese have become better at distracting themselves from upsetting stimuli and suppressing the external display of inner upset. In other words, young cosmopolitan Japanese have become more skillful at dissimulation and therefore less likely to fear blushing.

Eye contact may reveal one's thoughts and intentions, and it may also indicate prying concern with the inner states of one's companions. The deception of self and others reaches awareness on the level of discomfort surrounding eye contact. Tanishima Iwao, a Morita therapist, told me that though the Japanese traditionally used words to reveal themselves to others, they now use words to conceal themselves from others. Psychological discomfort from eye contact often indicates some level of deception and secrecy.

Turning next to consideration of the increase of neurotic depression, we find therapists who believe that this reaction is a response to realistic concerns in the lives of modern Japanese. According to some therapists, the fear that a single failure in life can affect one's whole future is perfectly valid under current conditions. It appears, for one, that choices of occupations or careers have become increasingly narrowed. Males in salaried positions specialize in their work to such a degree that at retirement they are unprepared to engage in other pursuits and activities; for example, they cannot cook and have not developed the habit of taking evening walks or talking with other family members. Therapists report a lack of self-sufficiency, a narrow self-image strongly tied to role specialization. Furthermore, there seems to be a basic inability to control or assure success; there is no way of assuring victory in the game of life even though one is playing well and hard. Thus, if the employer doesn't give a promotion or if the husband squanders money, there seems to be no effective recourse. Perhaps the picture painted here is harsher than reality; however, the sense of hopelessness and helplessness that accompanies neurotic depression becomes more understandable when considered in this light. Other depressive symptoms such as sleeplessness and lack of appetite may be associated with worries about repayment of loans, lack of job mobility and advancement, and the like.

Japanese Models of Psychotherapy

A definition is a conceptual tool more or less useful for a particular person or persons in a particular time and setting. In the next few sections we will consider some of the ways that a Japanese therapist and patient together come to define psychotherapy. Consideration of some models of Japanese therapy provide insights to such questions as: How do patients' conceptions of psychotherapy differ from those of their therapists? How does the training of therapists affect their definitions of therapy? How does a layperson learn to define psychotherapy, come to know what to expect from treatment, and evaluate which life problems require psychotherapeutic help? How does a patient's definition of psychotherapy change over time during therapy? How do therapists and patients negotiate to define or redefine the process and goals of therapy?

Four models or definitions of psychotherapy that are employed in Japan are presented below. For present purposes, psychotherapy is defined as a system of treatment for mental disturbance in which at least one variant of the system is practiced by physicians in hospitals. This definition excludes the mental health support and information offered through the media, friendships, educators, shamans, and so forth, but these dimensions often appear (usually implicitly) as underlying features of interactions between therapist and patient in Japan. The four models indicate implicit understandings of what psychotherapy constitutes in various settings. I have called them the healing model, the training model, the interaction model, and the salvation model. Each model posits a characteristic definition of the source of suffering, who may be suitable for treatment (and what that person is to be called), how treatment may proceed effectively, what constitutes cure or progress, and who has responsibility for that progress.

The Healing Model

Perhaps the most prevalent model of psychotherapy in modern Japan is the healing model. From this perspective, a patient goes to a therapist for relief from mental suffering just as an ill person seeks out a physician for cure of any disease symptom. This model implies some responsibility on the therapist's part for a correct diagnosis and an accurate prescription of medication, diet, and any other form of treatment deemed necessary. The patient, in return, must follow the therapist's directions faithfully. If by doing so relief is not forthcoming, the patient can change to another, more suitable therapist. Underlying this medical healing model is a consumer model. The therapist (usually a physician) offers a service. The patient knows what is the desired service and what is a satisfactory performance of the service. And the patient is free to shop around when the service is considered to be inferior. Chemotherapy provided by the general practitioner or psychiatrist fits this model well, as does behavior therapy and most hypnotherapies.

The Training Model

A second model found commonly within the practice of Japanese psychotherapies might broadly be called "training." From the perspective provided by this model, psychotherapy offers guidance for psychological growth and development. Like a tutor for college entrance examinations or a judo instructor or a teacher of flower arrangement, the psychotherapist provides information about aspects of living and advises the patient/trainee how to surmount lack of skill and ignorance.

The training model is quite different from that of the healing paradigm in that the tasks and goals of the participants are defined along different lines. In contrast with the healing model, in which the therapist is seen as the *chiryōsha* (medical healer), in the training model the therapist is viewed as a *shidōsha* (guide). As a guide, the therapist takes more responsibility in defining the patient's difficulties and progress. Within a healing framework the patient is the expert, basing judgments on current feeling states, because patients alone know best how they are feeling. However, within the training framework is the assumption that the trainee may not be mature enough to recognize the basic problem or the current status of progress. Feeling terrible, for example, may not be considered a misfortune of training but rather a marker in the trainee's development or an insignificant side effect of some much more important step forward into another area of growth.

The training therapist is responsible for shaping the regimen to fit the individual needs and stage of competency of the patient/trainee, but the trainee has final responsibility for progress. He or she must practice hard, devoting time and effort to self-development, demonstrating to the therapist commitment and a willingness to be shaped by the program. Failures in training therapies are never the fault of the therapist. Failures are always seen to be caused by the inadequate or misdirected efforts of the trainee. It follows that moving from teacher to teacher because of lack of progress makes little sense (in contrast with the consumerism of the healing model).

Morita therapy, some styles of Naikan, and Seiza therapy fit this model (Reynolds 1980). In less clear fashion it appears that Freudian therapy and transactional analysis are forced into this model by some Japanese patients. Zen trainees appear to operate with this conceptual model.

The Interaction Model

The interaction model is related to the training model and to the salvation model discussed below. The interaction model draws on the Japanese recognition of the importance of social relationships, and it is given additional support by the importance of the therapist-patient relationship in Western psychotherapeutic theory, which is held in high regard. In Japan, social ties such as those within families, work groups, and among classmates are generally strong and satisfying. It is understandable that a relationship, in this case the relationship between therapist and patient, can be seen to have a supporting, even a healing, quality. In the West, Rogerian and most psychoanalytic therapists stress the value of the therapist-patient relationship. In working with some neurotic and nearly all of the more severely disturbed patients, including psychiatric inpatients, most Japanese psychiatrists, psychologists, and social workers use this supportive mode of therapy.

The methods, goals, and mutual responsibilities of the interaction model of psychotherapy are ill defined. Again, the lack of adequate training in therapeutic techniques among those who practice in Japan must be emphasized. One of my Japanese therapist informants with extensive Western training pejoratively tagged this vague Japanese interaction style *"muntera,"* a term that means unskilled chatting. We must be careful here not to evaluate Japanese interaction therapy by some supposed Western standard. Patients do appreciate the attention and concern shown to them during therapeutic interactions. Doi (1973a) has pointed out the strong element of passive dependency *(amae)* in the Japanese character and the Japanese people's need for signals from others that they are being lovingly cared for. When therapists using interactional methods try to force self-revelation and openness into the therapeutic relationship (following culturally inappropriate Western guide-lines), they commonly encounter resistance from their Japanese patients. Severe problems have been reported in family therapy, T groups (face-to-face therapeutic groups focusing on interpersonal interaction), psycho-analysis, and encounter groups when too much pressure is exerted to reaffirm something other than positive, accepting interpersonal relation-ships.

The acceptance of Rogerian nondirective therapy by psychologists in Japan can be understood, in part by its lack of pressure in interaction. Japanese patients are very reluctant to express and merge *honne* and *tate-mae* (the personal / private and the socially acceptable / public aspects of self) even within a sheltered psychotherapeutic setting.

The interaction model implies a patient's unswerving trust in the ther-apist as an expert and mature human being. It also implies a long-term sustaining relationship—at least patients tend to infer such elements. Termination of therapy can be very difficult and complex and can bring with it feelings of abandonment. After all, family, classmates, and workmates are archetypes of long-term sustaining relationships. From the perspective of a newly admitted patient, it may appear unproductive to invest in a short-term therapeutic contact, no matter how supportive. In this model the therapist is less the healer or guide and more the dependable, strong, esteemed, and authoritative companion.

The Salvation Model

The final model for consideration here is religious, the model of salva-tion. Therapies in this mode offer two forms of relief from mental anguish. The first form is immediate. Relief comes when concerned advi-sors and fellow believers listen to the patient's tales of suffering and share their own experiences in return; the warmth of community acceptance and a sense of purposeful living envelop the patient. A unique form of long-term relief comes in the belief that suffering endured in the present will be vanquished in the world of life-after-death. Even though the validity of this promised relief cannot be ascertained before death ac-cording to any strictly rational standards of verification, the hope can nevertheless make current suffering more meaningful and more bear-able. Modern religious interpretations (in Buddhism and Christianity, for example) speak of heaven and hell in this life, thus focusing on changes of attitude and behavior in the here-and-now rather than in some afterlife. Naikan, one form of therapy that fits the salvation model, reflects this "terrafication" of religious concepts in its maxim "To act according to one's own convenience is to be a devil; to act according to the convenience of others is to be the Buddha." (It is interesting to note that somewhat secularized versions of Naikan are offered by physicians in hospitals in Kagoshima and on Honshu.)

Responsibility for salvation (not cure) within this model clearly lies in the devotee (not patient). Deities do not fail; human beings lack faith, perpetrate harmful acts, and fail to do good. Although efforts may be made by therapists to individualize the devotees' worship, the goal and means of salvation are absolute, following the scriptures. Ultimately, all must follow the same path to the same end.

Like the training model therapies, salvation therapies accept "normal" members as well as troubled ones. Similarly, both models tend to blur the boundaries between normal and abnormal. We are all ignorant, suffering, and in need of salvation.

Negotiation

I have suggested that Japanese patients perceive psychotherapy according to one or more of the four schemata presented above. Patients tend to select a mode of therapy that fits their perception of what psychotherapy ought to be. For example, a few years ago those who came for Naikan therapy at Gasshōen Temple in Mie prefecture tended to be elderly farm folk, strong believers in Jōdō Shinshū Buddhism, which, in stressing salvation, is congruent with the Gasshōen variant of Naikan. Such clients would have had a great deal of trouble adapting to a Freudian-based therapy. In contrast, those who attend the meetings of the Morita therapy mental health organization, Seikatsu no Hakkenkai, tend to be urban white-collar workers, young adults or of middle age. These meetings incorporate lectures and classroom discussion of assigned readings. The educational format of this style of Morita therapy echoes the past experiences of formal education in this middle-class population. It meets their current need for an intellectually understandable system taught within a formal educational context.

It is not realistic in the case of large, complex societies to assume that because therapist and client share the same basic cultural background they generally bring common notions, including models of therapy, to their encounter. Similarly, when therapist and client come from different cultural backgrounds, their therapy interaction will not necessarily be strained or fruitless (Reynolds and Kiefer 1977). Were there no social need for negotiation within the psychotherapy setting there would be no need for therapy itself. When the understanding of therapist and client match perfectly with a model and there is a shared commitment to that model, therapist and client are one. The exchange is something other than psychotherapy.

However, when a Japanese therapist perceives a client to be operating under assumptions of a model contradictory to the therapist's own views, there is usually some attempt to get the client to redefine assumptions so that both will operate similarly and congruently. My experience as a therapist in Japan and my observations of other therapists there have centered on situations in which therapists using training or salvation models encounter clients with contradictory healing models. The negotiations for reevaluation of the clients' problem, the process to bring about improvement in the condition, and the criteria of progress are of great interest. What takes place during these negotiations? Although studies are still incomplete, I can offer some preliminary thoughts and observations.

In this area of redefinition, one of the first tasks for the therapist is to establish an image of having an expertise and specific knowledge regarding the client's case. This image enhances the therapist's bargaining power in reaching agreement with the client on the model of therapy. The therapist's expertise can be established by certain titles and educational degrees and by publication of books and pamphlets describing cured patients with problems like those of the negotiating client. Successes in therapy and testimonies may also be paraded during meetings attended by previously treated clients and newcomers, and the therapist may point to self-cure using the preferred method.

In Morita therapy the therapist often asks questions that are, in fact, predictions about the client's symptoms. For example, the therapist might ask, "And, then, after you became self-conscious about looking into people's eyes while carrying on a conversation, didn't you begin to fear that other people recognized that you were self-conscious?" Once the client is convinced that the therapist truly understands his or her problems, an important step has been achieved in model bargaining.

It is rare to hear a therapist ridicule, interrupt, or flatly contradict a client's choice of therapy model. Rather, the therapist listens politely, then attempts some variety of reeducation. It may be useful to have other, more advanced clients teach the preferred model to newcomers. In inpatient Morita therapy this task is accomplished through meetings and group living, and in the Moritist mental health organization, through group meetings, retreats, and magazine articles about personal experiences. In Naikan therapy extensive use is made of audio tapes of prior clients' insights. These tapes, which are broadcast over an intercom system in many Naikan facilities, provide models of proper introspection, insight, and the preferred view of therapy to later Naikan clients.

Through the influence of the therapist, fellow clients, and written and audio materials, the client comes to reinterpret ongoing and past experiences as more in accord with the preferred model. At Kora Kōseiin, for example, the client comes to adopt the Moritist perspective that living a full life in spite of suffering is more important than relief from suffering. The healing model that the client may earlier have held is now abandoned. At Gasshōen the client learns how to use suffering as encouragement to purify the heart, a goal more worthy than immediate relief of symptoms. Again, the healing model is abandoned. Both Morita therapy and Naikan teach the client that relief from suffering may occur, but such relief is merely a by-product of the more important task of character development.

Typically, when negotiations fail, the client struggles and struggles but eventually searches for another therapist whose style better fits his or her initial model. To continue in therapy with an incongruent model is to engage in a meaningless and painful exercise. A few clients continue with the original therapist, trusting the character of the therapist but failing to adopt the therapist's model. By definition, there can be no satisfactory resolution of the client's difficulties in such situations because the models include divergent definitions of "resolution."

Common Features

Thus far we have considered primarily differences among four models of Japanese psychotherapy. There are, however, some fundamental features that are employed in nearly every form of therapy in Japan. These common features provide a clue to the essential ingredients of any successful therapy as well as insight into the essence of neurotic disorder.

One feature common to most forms of therapy is specification. The practice of requiring the patient to be specific, detailed, and precise in descriptions of self and symptoms is a key element to successful therapy. The intake interview of the various therapies requires such specification and can be viewed as part of the therapy process, not merely as a precursor to therapy. Morita and Naikan therapists ask for detailed accounts of the symptoms, when they began, specific problems resulting from them, and the like. Psychoanalysis calls for detailed specification of dreams and other material from the productions of the client's mind. Within the framework of salvation therapies, vague confessions are unsatisfactory; they must be detailed and precise.

The neurotic person characteristically tries to escape from these demands for specification by making abstract, vague, ambiguous, generalized statements. "I've always been this way." "I felt terrible all week." "Nobody ever liked me." Such statements are characteristic of the neurotic person's estrangement from everyday concrete reality. Concreteness and precise specification force the client to think in more realistic terms about self and world.

A second characteristic of neurotics is a sort of self-centeredness, an aspect of neurosis that is noted and dealt with by Japanese therapeutic systems by techniques to dissolve self-focus. The clients focus attention on what is happening to them, to their feelings, tensions, and problems. Morita therapists point out that this self-focus prevents the client from observing reality, what is actually occurring at any given moment. Accordingly, self-centeredness restricts the client's ability to respond realistically, to merge the self with the immediate situation. Naikan therapists see this inflated self-centeredness as a sort of screen that obscures the clients' perception of who they really are—takers from others more than givers and sources of trouble and burdens to those around them. When the clients come to an experimental understanding of who they are (through Naikan introspection), feelings of contrition and gratitude will emerge and the self-focus will be redirected toward serving significant others.

It is worth noting that many Japanese (and Western) psychotherapies seek to dissolve this excessive self-focus through initial flooding of the client with an excess of self-focus. Absolute bed rest in Morita therapy, Naikan meditation, Shadan therapy, *zazen* (sitting Zen meditation), *seiza* (a form of quiet sitting meditation with emphasis on proper breathing), free association in psychoanalysis, baseline recording and step construction in behavior therapy, systematic desensitization, reflecting techniques in Rogerian therapy—all focus the clients' attention on themselves as the initial step in eventually pulling their attention away from the neurotic self-focus.

A third feature common to all therapies is the requirement that the client do something. The sort of doing varies, of course, from therapy to therapy. In some forms the doing is meditation (focused attention) or work therapy or talking for long periods or taking medication. Even within the context of medication, the therapeutic interaction often centers on when and where and whether or not the client consistently takes the prescribed medication. In other words, no therapy allows the clients simply to be totally passive; some responsible effort on their part is required. Like the dissolution of self-focus, such tactics pull the client back into dealing with everyday reality.

Another feature common to all therapies is the use of the weight of authority. It struck me as I watched a recent Japanese television serial based on the famous tale of the forty-seven samurai that the hated Lord Kira was consistently referred to in honorific terms, even by his avowed enemies. He was Kira-*dono* and Kira-*sama* (terms reflecting his high position), but never the Japanese equivalents of "that Kira" or "the dog Kira" or even the ordinary Japanese equivalent of "Mr. Kira." He automatically deserved use of proper exalted terms of address and reference simply because he was a member of the nobility.

My informants report (and my observations confirm) that there is no such perfect consistency in following this custom today (if, in fact, there was in the past). Nevertheless, compared with Americans, modern Japanese speakers do tend to use verbal markers of high status based on social position (and not on some personal relationship or mood of the speaker) when addressing or referring to persons of social status markedly higher than their own. Americans appear generally to use nonstatus referents to social superiors when not in their presence. Similarly, Americans seem more likely to shift estimations of the debts they owe parents on the basis of fluctuations in their personal feelings about their parents at the moment. It is not uncommon during my research in gerontology to see elderly Americans desperately try to avoid arguments and maintain smooth relations with their offspring in order to assure themselves of continued affection and economic support. Such circumstances are not unknown in Japan, but I encounter them less frequently there.

One principle underlying these patterns of behavior is that social status carries more weight than temporary feelings *(kimochi)* in Japan than in the United States. Authority has enjoyed particular privilege in Japan, as is to be expected from a *tate shakai,* a society with strong vertical organization.

In the light of this traditional respect for authority it is useful to note recent trends of rebelliousness toward institutionalized positions of authority and the orientation of indigenous psychotherapies toward issues of authority. Newspapers and television news broadcasts are filled with reports on intrafamily violence (children attacking parents), intra-school violence (students attacking teachers), lawbreaking (drug traffic, homicide, burglary, embezzlement), legal action against corporations and public figures, and demonstrations against the military and against the country itself. It is not difficult to think that these news items reflect an explosive challenge to authority within the family, schools, laws, business, government, the military, and even toward the hallowed national identity.

Challenges to authority may be understood (if not always condoned) in terms of individual and personal feelings and assessments of immediate situations. Authority in and of itself is no longer sufficient to ensure deference. In the past, challenges to authority in Japan were usually couched in self-sacrificial behavior such as suicide on the doorstep of a politician. Modern challenges may involve some risk but often hold the possibility of immediate reward as well. This modern-day defiance is regarded by some as a reaction to uncritical acceptance of the demands of authority and a move toward healthy disrespect and critical doubting of social power—along American cultural lines. However it is viewed, it is clear that authority in Japan faces assault on many fronts. What have Japanese Buddhist-based therapies such as Morita therapy and Naikan to say about authority, and what can they offer the modern client pulled about by shifting tides of authority and challenge in modern Japan?

It can be argued that a major element of all Japanese psychotherapies involves a restructuring of attitudes toward authority figures and a subsequent refocus of the client's thoughts toward therapeutic issues. The model and representative of authority within the psychotherapy setting is, of course, the therapist. What therapy offers the client in orientation toward authority will be reflected in the relationship between therapist and client. In Morita therapy the therapist remains a strong leader with overt directive influence tempered by paternalistic concern, much like the traditional pattern. In this setting, however, the authority figure is seen to have suffered, too. The therapists are very likely to relate their own experiences of neurotic misery before their encounters with Morita's method. This facilitates patient identification with this authority figure. Identification makes more palatable therapists' authority to regulate their patients' lives. It also prompts patients to endure the strict regimen by offering hope that they can overcome suffering, just as their therapists did. The refocusing element of therapy involves the shift toward having patients see their own responsibility in governing their lives moment by moment. Without relying on authority to direct them, they must learn to discover what needs to be done in this moment and in the next. Authority is taken for granted, but personal initiative is stressed.

In Naikan, both within the setting itself and in guided reflection on the past, the client is presented with images of authority figures who are kind and supportive regardless of the client's faults. Therapists will suggest particular meditation themes during each visit, thus directing their clients course of therapy, but the therapists will also bow to clients and serve them food, listen patiently to their confessions, and offer encouragement or even shed a tear with them. Again, the authority of the therapist remains unchallenged, taken for granted. Unlike Morita therapy, where the therapist's authority is buttressed with the sense that straightforward directing is required in that setting in those moments, Naikan encourages clients to view the therapist's authority as a kind of service, as what the client needs. Both elements, authoritarian guidance and personal initiative, are present in both therapies, but the emphasis seems different. In Naikan, refocusing of attention directs the clients to evaluate what they did in their relationships with others (particularly authority figures). They are encouraged to ask themselves what they contributed to their superiors, what troubles they caused authority figures. Again, the acceptance of the "natural" system of authority is balanced by a recognition of personal responsibility and meaningfulness of action.

Neither Morita therapy nor Naikan supports feelings of impotence in the client. Both refocus the clients' attention toward the ways in which the clients themselves influence the world, all the while accepting the influence of authority over them. Because all human beings must come to terms with reality of powerful figures in their lives from infancy through adulthood, these Japanese methods (and the resulting attitudes toward authority) are worth consideration as resolutions of these panhuman issues.

A final shared feature of therapies worth mentioning here is the initial acceptance of clients as they are. For the therapist to do otherwise would be to risk causing the client to leave the therapy setting, or, possibly, to sabotage the therapy process. Although not always explicitly verbalized each therapist has in mind a model of what humans are, what neurosis is, what cure is, and why clients are as they are (London 1964). As we have seen, this model may not be identical to the models that clients bring to therapy. Yet therapy must start somewhere, and it starts with acceptance, not rejection, of the clients themselves. Though a particular client's model of therapy may be rejected ultimately, the psychotherapist sets an example by accepting the client as a person. Such an example may eventually help the clients to accept themselves.

Final Thoughts

In this overview of Japanese approaches to mental health I have emphasized the socially legitimized variations. As in the United States, in addition to formal therapeutic systems there are numerous informal and religious methods of dealing with mental health problems. Even within recognized psychotherapeutic institutions and clinics there are fads and regional variations. What I have presented appears, necessarily, more systematic than is the case in actual practice.

Two of the therapeutic systems described above, Morita and Naikan therapy, have been introduced to the West with some initial success. It remains to be seen whether Japanese therapies will have a major impact on treatment methods in the West.

References

Bowers, J. Z. 1965. *Medical education in Japan.* New York: Harper and Row.
Caudill, W. 1976. The cultural and interpersonal context of everyday health and illness in Japan and America. In *Asian medical systems,* ed. C. Leslie. Berkeley and Los Angeles: Univ. of California Press.
Caudill, W., and C. Schooler. 1969. Symptom patterns and background characteristics of Japanese psychiatric patients. In *Mental health research in Asia and the Pacific,* ed. W. Caudill and T. Lin. Honolulu: East-West Center Press.
DeVos, G. 1973. *Socialization for achievement.* Berkeley and Los Angeles: Univ. of California Press.
———. 1980. Afterword. In D. K. Reynolds, *The quiet therapies.* Honolulu: Univ. of Hawaii Press.
Doi, T. 1973a. *The anatomy of dependence.* Tokyo: Kodansha.
———. 1973b. *Omote* and *ura. Journal of Nervous and Mental Disease* 157 (4): 258–261.
———. 1978. *Seishin ryōhō ni shinpo wa aru ka* (Is there progress in psychotherapy?) *Rinshō Seishin Igaku* 8 (6): 627–629.

Draguns, J. G., et al. 1971. Symptomatology of hospitalized psychiatric patients in Japan and the United States. *Journal of Nervous and Mental Disease* 152:3–16.

Fujinawa, A., and Y. Kasahara. 1973. The psychiatric experience of having self or part of self escaping into the external world. In *World biennial of psychiatry and psychotherapy.* New York: Basic Books.

Ikegami, N. 1980. Growth of psychiatric beds in Japan. *Social Science and Medicine* 14A:561–570.

Ikemi, Y., and M. Sugita. 1975. The Oriental version of transactional analysis. *Psychosomatics* 16:164–169.

Iwai, H., and D. K. Reynolds. 1970. Morita therapy. *American Journal of Psychiatry* 126 (7): 1031–1036.

Jones, W. T. 1976. World views and Asian medical systems. In *Asian medical systems,* ed. C. Leslie. Berkeley and Los Angeles: Univ. of California Press.

Kato, M. 1969. Psychiatric epidemiological surveys in Japan. In *Mental health research in Asia and the Pacific,* ed. W. Caudill and T. Lin. Honolulu: East-West Center Press.

Kitsuse, J. I. 1965. Moral treatment and reformation of inmates in Japanese prisons. *Psychologia* 8:9–23.

Kondo, A. 1953. Morita therapy. *American Journal of Psychoanalysis* 13:31–37.

Kora, Y. 1965. Morita therapy. *International Journal of Psychiatry* 1 (4): 611–640.

Kora, T., and K. Ohara. 1973. Morita therapy. *Psychology Today* 6 (10): 63–68.

Kumasaka, Y., and S. Yoshioka. 1968. The law of private imprisonment. *American Journal of Psychiatry* 125:109–112.

London, P. 1964. *The modes and morals of psychotherapy.* New York: Holt, Rinehart and Winston.

Maruyama, S., et al. 1982. Taijinkyōfu no jidaiteki hensen (Historical changes in phobias concerning interpersonal relations). *Seishin Igaku* 11:37–43.

Morita, S. 1983. *Seishin ryōhō kōgi* (Psychotherapy lectures). Tokyo: Hakuyosha.

Murase, T. 1974. Naikan therapy. In *Japanese culture and behavior,* ed. T. Lebra and W. Lebra. Honolulu: Univ. of Hawaii Press.

Ohara, K., and D. K. Reynolds. 1968. Changing methods in Morita psychotherapy. *International Journal of Social Psychiatry* 14 (4): 305–310.

Reynolds, D. K. 1976. *Morita psychotherapy.* Berkeley and Los Angeles: Univ. of California Press.

———. 1977. Naikan therapy—an experimental view. *International Journal of Social Psychiatry* 23 (4): 252–264.

———. 1980. *The quiet therapies.* Honolulu: Univ. of Hawaii Press.

———. 1981a. Morita psychotherapy. In *Handbook of innovative psychotherapies,* ed. R. Corsini. New York: Wiley.

———. 1981b. Naikan therapy. In *Handbook of innovative psychotherapies,* ed. R. Corsini. New York: Wiley.

———. 1981c. Psychocultural perspectives on death. In *Living and dying with cancer,* ed. P. Ahmed. New York: Elsevier.

———. 1983. *Naikan psychotherapy.* Chicago: Univ. of Chicago Press.

———. 1984a. *Constructive living.* Honolulu: Univ. of Hawaii Press.

———. 1984b. *Playing ball on running water.* New York: W. Morrow.

Reynolds, D. K., and C. W. Kiefer. 1977. Cultural adaptability as an attribute of therapies. *Culture, Medicine and Psychiatry* 1:395–412.

Reynolds, D. K., and J. Yamamoto. 1972. East meets West. *Science and Psychoanalysis* 21:187–193.

———. 1973. Morita psychotherapy in Japan. *Current Psychiatric Therapies* 13:219–227.

Rin, H., C. Schooler, and W. Caudill. 1973. Symptomatology and hospitalization. *Journal of Nervous and Mental Disease* 157:296–312.

Sakamoto, Y. 1976. Some experiences through family psychotherapy for psychotics in Japan. *International Journal of Social Psychiatry* 22:265–271.

Sasaki, Y. 1969a. Non-medical healing in contemporary Japan. In *Culture bound syndromes, ethnopsychiatry, and alternate therapies,* ed. W. Lebra. Honolulu: Univ. of Hawaii Press, an East-West Center Book.

———. 1969b. Psychiatric study of the shaman in Japan. In *Mental health research in Asia and the Pacific,* ed. W. Caudill and T. Lin. Honolulu: East-West Center Press.

Suzuki, T., and R. Suzuki. 1977. Morita therapy. In *Psychosomatic medicine,* ed. E. D. Wittkower and H. Warnes. New York: Harper and Row.

———. 1981. The effectiveness of in-patient Morita therapy. *Psychiatric Quarterly* 53 (3): 201–213.

Takeuchi, K. 1965. On Naikan. *Psychologia* 8:2–8.

Terashima, S. 1969. The structure of rejecting attitudes toward the mentally ill in Japan. In *Mental health research in Asia and the Pacific,* ed. W. Caudill and T. Lin. Honolulu: East-West Center Press.

Yamaguchi, T., and A. Yamaguchi. 1973. Permissiveness and psychotherapy in Japan. *Journal of Nervous and Mental Disease* 157 (4): 292–295.

Yamamoto, Kazuo. 1972. A comparative study of patienthood in Japanese and American mental hospitals. In *Transcultural research in mental health,* ed. W. Lebra. Honolulu: Univ. of Hawaii Press, an East-West Center Book.

Yokoyama, K. 1968. Morita therapy and Seiza. *Psychologia* 11 (3–4): 179–184.

Protests of a Good Wife and Wise Mother: The Medicalization of Distress in Japan

MARGARET LOCK

The great strategies of power encrust themselves
and depend for their conditions of exercise on the
level of the micro-relations of power.
—Michel Foucault, *Power-Knowledge*

A visit to the health-related book section of any reasonably well-stocked bookstore in Japan today leaves one with the impression that here is a nation bent on educating itself in preventive medicine, self-care, self-diagnosis, and the correct selection of appropriate professionally supplied therapeutic alternatives. A large proportion of the books are variations of what is known as *katei no igaku* (family medicine). Such books furnish up-to-the-minute accounts of basic physiology and anatomy, of first aid, and of the contemporary symptomatology, diagnosis, and treatment of all but the most rare of diseases. For those who use traditional techniques in addition to biomedicine, there is a shiny new volume on the modern application of herbal medicine, acupuncture, moxibustion, and massage. These books are usually published by respectable and apparently neutral sources such as the Japanese Broadcasting Corporation and the Asahi and the Mainichi newspapers, and they are often a gift of the local government to residents of certain cities as part of preventive medicine promotion campaigns. Such books are the culmination of a long tradition of publications related to self-care in Japan, and they shore up an old value: that individuals and primary groups are basically responsible for the maintenance of health and the occurrence of illness.

Apart from the "home doctor" and "family medicine" books, there is a large selection of medically related volumes written mostly by doctors but also by journalists. A quick perusal of the titles and chapter headings immediately excites an anthropologically trained reader, since they provide evidence that culture-bound syndromes are proliferating in modern

Japan. Titles include mention of the kitchen syndrome, moving-day depression, child-rearing neurosis, refusal-to-go-to-school syndrome, and so on. Other titles use names that North Americans are more familiar with: hypochondriasis, hysteria, sleep disorders, impotence, hyperactivity, and anorexia. But even when labels are focused on this more psychophysiological level, there are some surprises, such as "disharmony of the autonomic nervous system."

The "medicalization of life," as Illich calls it, is clearly rampant in Japan. Medicalization is usually depicted in the literature as a process in which the medical community attempts to create a "market" for its services by redefining as diseases certain events, behavior, and problems (see, for example, Freidson 1970; Illich 1976; MacPherson 1981; Merkin 1976; Szasz 1970; Zola 1978). The institution of medicine is seen as serving the interests of powerful controlling groups in a society; in Zola's words it is "a major institution of control . . . nudging aside law and religion" in which ordinary people lose their rights of control and autonomy over their own lives. Zola believes that this tendency is reinforced by the haste with which many people bring everyday troubles to the care and attention of the doctor.

Studies on medicalization have been criticized most frequently for their apparent lack of attention to the fact that the institution and practice of medicine itself reflects the structure of the society in question. Medicine therefore serves to express and reinforce the social relations of the larger society including those of class, race, sex, and age (see, for example, Ehrenreich 1978; Frankenberg 1980; Krause 1977; Stark 1982; Waitzkin and Waterman 1974; Young 1982). The incidence of disease and illness is reflected in these same social relations, but when physical disorder is conceptualized as either a biological or a personal problem it serves to divert attention from the larger social issues involved.

One of the tasks of the anthropologist is to explore how physical illness, which frequently serves as a symbolic representation of social and interpersonal conflict, is dealt with by ordinary people and by professionals, how its management reproduces the values of society at large, and how the original conflict is or is not resolved in the process.

In the West, one response to the recent barrage of criticism against biomedicine has been the emergence of the holistic health movement, which encourages self-responsibility in connection with health and illness. Guttmacher (1979, 16) points out the advantages of this viewpoint but hastens to add that by seeing health as an end in itself and by emphasizing individual responsibility the movement has in fact exacerbated the medicalization of many areas of life and reinforced a basic biomedical premise: that disorders should be dealt with largely at the personal level. Guttmacher adds that this attitude receives government support since it is equated with cost containment.

In Japan, there is an even stronger tendency than in North America to reify health, to consider it a personal or often family problem, and to rush to the doctor for medication and psychological support. The roots of this behavior can be found in traditional East Asian medicine (Lock 1980) and indigenous psychotherapeutic systems (Reynolds 1980) as well as associated philosophical and religious systems, all of which are active today and enjoying revived support. The mass media has recently coined the phrase *kenkō-būmu* (health boom) to describe the burgeoning interest in natural food. This, together with the vast popular medical literature, attests to a keen public interest and sense of personal responsibility for health and illness.

In this chapter I discuss forms of protest in Japan, including the somatization of distress, especially in women. Some approaches to the management of somatization by the medical profession in contemporary Japan are considered. An attempt is made to show how these approaches are influenced in part by a belief in science and technology, at times by the self-interest of the medical profession and, in addition, by ideas of long standing about self-responsibility for health and illness. Management of somatization is also influenced by shared ideas about acceptable modes for the expression of conflict and, in connection with female patients, by current ideas about the nature of women and the family. The medical system and medicalization, however, act not only as mirrors of social organization and cultural beliefs, but also potentially as vehicles for social change. Biomedicine is not a monolithic organization, even within one society, nor is it a single systematized form of medical practices and beliefs. At the level of physician-patient interaction, it represents a perpetual reworking of changing values, new knowledge, and new technology (Gaines and Hahn 1985). It most frequently appears to act as a force for conservatism and, at times, of repression, but since its basic business is the management of suffering and pain, which by its very nature raises questions of ambiguity and paradox, it can also act as a stimulus for the creation of new meanings, and hence social action. In the following pages I also try to show how in the process of medicalization private distress and suffering become public knowledge and are exposed to scrutiny. This process, therefore, can serve potentially to instigate an awareness of the "hegemonic" forms of certain social institutions (Gramsci 1971) and hence sow the seeds for change, in this case in the status in women.

"Soft Rule": Japanese Concepts of Power

A well-known Japanese intellectual historian, Kamishima Jiro, distinguishes Japanese sociopolitical development, which he describes as an "assimilating unitary society," from typical Western development, which he labels as an "alienizing composite society." He believes that much of Western history is based upon a pattern of conquest and subjugation of people that sets up situations of conflict and a questioning of political authority. In contrast, until World War II Japan had never been overrun in historic times. As a consequence its culture has developed by absorbing and assimilating things from the outside, by "making the strange familiar" (Kamishima 1973, 8).

Georg Simmel (1969) claims that for people to develop a clear conception of political authority and thereby to demystify it, they must have experience of more than one kind of authority; only thus can they learn that authority is not part of an inalienable natural order. Koschmann (1978), drawing on the work of Bellah (1962), Harootunian (1974), and Kamishima (1973), among many others, demonstrates how the "givenness" of authority is reflected in Japanese religious and ethical traditions and reaffirmed through linguistic domains such as the distinction between *watakushi* (I or me) and *oyake* (the public). In the Meiji era (1868–1912), for example, *oyake* was always associated with high-sounding purpose: public tranquility and order, fairness, and the "consultation of public opinion" *(kōgi)*. *Watakushi* was identified with irregular dealings, bad faith, selfishness, personal feelings, and private desires. In the inevitable encounter between the public and personal realms, individuals were admonished, as a kind of moral imperative, "to dissolve the personal and honor the public *(messhi hōkō)*" (Harootunian 1974).

The actual exercise of power in Japan has been characterized as "soft rule," in which the preservation of harmony and suppression of conflict takes priority over individual rights and needs. Koschmann (1978, 19) states that "when oppression is soft and persuasive, feelings of dependency and relatedness persevere to obscure the irreducible atom of individuality and perpetuate the belief that what is real is to be found outside the individual, *between* himself and others rather than within." Psychological studies carried out in contemporary Japan reinforce this conclusion (DeVos 1973, 144; Doi 1973).

The Expression of Resistance

In a social system such as Japan's, forms of resistance to the all-enveloping cloak of authority are not usually those of open conflict, which are in any case disparaged, but tend to be less direct (see White 1984 for some notable exceptions to this pattern). Tsurumi (1974), a sociologist using historical and contemporary sources, concludes that two types of resistance, "retreatism" and "ritualism," are frequently used in Japan. The tradition of voluntary or forced separation from the community (retreatism) is called *yamairi* (entering the mountains) and was traditionally used to imply permanent seclusion. A 1975 survey (Murray 1975) estimated that ninety thousand contemporary Japanese had voluntarily undergone *ningen jōhatsu* ("human evaporation," that is, they had completely vanished). These people had apparently chosen retreatism as a form of protest. The second form of resistance, ritualism, involves the preservation inside oneself of nonconformist values while at the same time outwardly conforming with established behavior patterns. Koschmann (1978, 20) states that "ritualism means the preservation internally of contradiction. It implies accommodation within the personality of mutually contradictory elements (including values, belief systems, emotional responses) rather than their external expression and resolution through conflict." Japanese society as a whole can best be viewed as pluralistic or having multiple layers of value orientations and ideology (Bellah 1957; Lock 1980), and Tsurumi (1972) characterizes both Japanese social structure and Japanese personality as multilayered; the psychological mechanisms of suppression and not repression appear to be dominant.

Ritualistic resistance is probably the usual form of protest in Japan. Like retreatism, it does not lead directly to reform or social change. There are two characteristic styles of ritualistic resistance. The first, more common mode is institutionalized or "orderly" conflict. This is conflict acted out "in a predictable manner (often implicitly expected and accepted by the adversary) primarily for the purpose of symbolically affirming the separate interests, identities, and goals of the participants" (Krauss, Rohlen, and Steinhoff 1984, 9). The best-known example is the annual "spring labor offensive," during which the national unions go on strike for a prearranged day or two. Such ritualized resistance avoids direct confrontation and is not designed to bring about major changes in institutional structures but rather serves to remind everyone involved that there are ground rules to be observed.

The second type involves a dramatic self-sacrifice, often by one or more individuals who usually know that their goals are unattainable but who nevertheless choose to demonstrate sincerity of purpose and purity of motive. This form of resistance is frequently expressed through ritual suicide. The cases of Mishima Yukio and Okamoto Kozo (of the Red Army) are two of the best-known recent examples. Rather than trying to implement social change directly through organized, instrumental action, such protest is designed to create "symbolic affirmation of [one's] own principles" (Krauss 1974, 111) and, in addition, to try to incite one's antagonists to action by inducing guilt in them (DeVos, 1973, 472).

Not only at the level of group conflict, but also in cases of interpersonal conflict, nonconfrontational tactics are considered more appropriate than an outward, abrupt shattering of the peace. Lebra (1984b, 41) identifies seven strategies that are resorted to with regularity in potentially tense situations. One strategy is anticipatory management. Negative communication, that is, remaining silent when a response could be expected, is another. A third tactic is situational code switching, in which people who are in discord in one situation can be cooperative in other situations. Open confrontation may also be avoided by triadic management, in which a third party is resorted to as a go-between to aid negotiations. The strategy of displacement occurs when a disgruntled party, acting consciously or unconsciously, complains indirectly by stating that a third party rather than themselves is dissatisfied or by complaining to a third party or by expressing dissatisfaction through the mediumship of the ancestors or the spirit world (see also Yoshida 1984, 85). The sixth strategy, that of acceptance, represents a fatalistic resignation to an unsatisfactory state of affairs and is well documented as characteristic of Japanese behavior (Lebra 1974). The final nonconfrontational tactic commonly manifested in situations of discord is self-aggression, which can take the form of belittling oneself, expressing inadequacy or, in extreme cases, committing suicide. This last tactic, the interpersonal version of ritualistic resistance, is usually associated with the induction of guilt in others, especially if those others perceive themselves as the cause of suffering. I believe that somatization often represents a special but common case of self-aggression. As a form of protest, somatization, like other types of self-aggression, may often be unconscious, or only partly conscious; but, nevertheless, like ritual suicide, it can represent an attempt to induce changes in the behavior of the people affecting one's life.

Somatization and Interpersonal Relations

Somatization can best be defined as "both the expression of physical complaints in the absence of defined organic pathology and the amplification of symptoms resulting from established physical pathology (e.g., chronic disease)" (Kleinman 1982, 129). It has been hypothesized that whether one uses predominantly psychological or physiological modes for the expression of distress depends upon two major determinants: "actual adult experiences with symptoms and illness on the one hand, and cultural influences on the definition of illness on the other. Whereas reporting physical symptoms is culturally more neutral, reporting psychological symptoms is more dependent on social acceptability" (Mechanic 1980, 154).

Research carried out by both anthropologists and physicians indicates that the body is habitually used symbolically as a vehicle for expressing stress and oppression. The form that the expression takes is culturally constructed and can range from a dramatized performance or ritual, to the employment of altered states of consciousness, to direct verbalization of the problem, through to more subtle forms in which the corporeal body rebels. These symbolic representations can also be interpreted in a more constructive light, not only as an "idiom of distress" but as a plea for help, for change, for release from drudgery or humiliation (Comaroff 1982; Comaroff 1985; Devisch 1985; Good 1977; Helman 1985; Lewis 1971; Lock 1986; Mechanic 1980; Minuchin, Baker, and Rosman 1978; Nichter 1981). Kleinman, after reviewing recent research on the topic, stresses that somatization need not necessarily result from or represent psychopathology; it might be regarded as a particular "cognitive-behavioral type" with adaptive or maladaptive consequences that involve assessment of particular social and cultural as much as personal variables (1982, 130).

In Japan several aspects of the cultural heritage in addition to the attitudes toward conflict described above serve to reinforce a tendency to somatize. The form that interpersonal relations and their related language takes is important and so, too, are ideas derived from the Confucian and the Buddhist heritage.

Interpersonal Relations and the Expression of Needs

Every society appears to make some distinction between ideal and actual behavior, but the Japanese language employs several dichotomies that indicate to what a fine art this discrimination can be developed. For example, one situation is distinguished from another according to whether it is defined as *uchi* (in, inside, internal, private, us) or *soto* (out, outside, external, public, them), and one modifies one's behavior accordingly. But these distinctions are not fixed; they are, rather, fluid categories, socially relative, and dependent, for example, upon whether one is dealing with another individual, one's family, a Japanese company, or a foreign company.

There is a second dichotomy, that of *tatemae* and *honne*, which refers not so much to social expectations, as do the above categories, but more to one's personal intentions. Whereas *honne* means one's real or true intentions, *tatemae* refers to the principles that one should act by. These two concepts represent a source of conflict that all individuals everywhere face, but the emphasis in Japanese culture is upon the indirect expression or even suppression of *honne* for the sake of smooth interpersonal relations.

Formal behavior is based upon the notions of *tatemae* and *soto* (outside), which are close to the concept of a persona. Much of daily behavior in the home, school, or at work is the formal type of behavior, in which speech styles, gestures, and postures reinforce the nature of social relations between the people involved. Certain regions of Japan are known to express less *honne* than others. The mayor of Osaka said recently that the difference between Tokyo and Osaka is that Tokyo is more *tatemae* while Osaka is more *honne*. Not only is there geographical variation in the expression of *honne*, there is also variation due to status and role. In general, men, especially elderly men, can express *honne* most easily and acceptably. Women, usually both within and outside the home, should not express *honne*, although when alone with female relatives or close friends they may release their feelings (hence the importance in traditional life of wellside gossip and the public bath).

If during most of a person's daily life the direct expression of emotions and needs is frowned upon, other forms of expression become adaptive. Somatization, in addition to the other nonconfrontational tactics described above, is one such adaptive technique. It is acceptable to talk about tiredness, pain, dizzyness, palpitations, being languid, having tingling sensations, and so on ad nauseum and then to manipulate (often unconsciously) the behavior of others as they respond to the distress that is being expressed. Somatization and the presentation of non-specific complaints are frequent reasons for visits to the doctor's office in Japan (Lock 1980; Reynolds 1976; Vogel 1978), and an examination of their meaning to patients and physicians as well as their management can provide insights into the process and justification for medicalization. These insights serve in turn to highlight those situations and relationships in Japanese society that are often associated with conflict, distress, and ambiguity.

Interpreting and Managing Illness

There has never been a split between psyche and soma in Japanese thinking. Both physicians and patients readily attribute nonspecific somatic complaints, symptoms of depression *(yūutsu)* and other "psychosomatic" symptomatology to stress. An exploration of the principal factors contributing to stress will usually lead rapidly to concern about relationships within the family or at work. But this concern is generally expressed in an abstract or neutral fashion and only rarely will patients in a clinical setting make a direct statement about their personal situation or feelings. The restraints of formal behavior and communication, reinforced by Confucian mores, do not allow the expression of what is *uchi* (in this case, within the family). Illness and somatization are interpreted as expressions of stress at the social level, but since harmony is highly valued and the forms of social behavior and distribution of power cannot easily be questioned (and take primacy over the individual), the individual is expected to adjust so that harmony is restored. The first resort, therefore, is to medication in order to assist in this adjustment. The majority of physicians and patients believe that if physical order is restored, then, since psyche and soma are indivisible, emotional balance and social harmony will return as well. Family members, employers, and friends can be very patient and supportive during this process, and insurance companies allow long periods of hospitalization (Lock 1980). The ultimate objective of taking medication is not to provide relief of symptoms (although this is naturally welcome) but to facilitate reintegration into one's social role.

Use of nonverbal and nonconfrontational forms of communication reflect and are reinforced not only by Confucian mores but also by the Buddhist heritage, which gives high priority to inductive, intuitive, and experiential forms of learning. Buddhism encourages the view that verbal interaction is a form of communication obviously necessary to cope with daily life but incapable of fully expressing the complexity of one's inner state, which is better not revealed, or only partially revealed through thoughtful action (Lebra 1976, 46; Reynolds 1980).

Responsibility for Health and Healing

Illness represents disorder, and the activities and explanations that people use to deal with illness are an attempt to restore order and control. Medical activities and knowledge, both lay and professional, are shaped by their cultural context (Good 1977; Kleinman 1979; Lock 1980), and the core values that provide a sense of coherence to an individual's life are also relied upon in attempts to interpret and attribute meaning to illness. These same values are drawn upon to structure relationships between physicians and patients, and patients and their families.

Explanations about the causes of illness and misfortune have implications for the allocation of responsibility in connection with the occurrence of the events. It is characteristic of the medical systems of nonliterate societies (those using externalizing discourses, in Young's terms [1976]) to locate the causes of illness outside of the sick person's body, in important events leading up to an illness episode, and in so doing they tap religious beliefs, kin relationships, and economic and political alignments. By explaining the causes of illness in this way, the occurrence of illness is associated with morality and norms of conduct. In medical systems (such as the traditional system of Japan) that use theories of balance and homeostasis as their basis, individual and family responsibility for the preservation of balance is considered important. The occurrence of illness in this type of medical system is not associated so much with immorality as with irresponsibility and neglect. In the biomedical system the incidence of illness is theoretically interpreted as a neutral event (Habermas 1971); but, due partly to the critical scrutiny biomedicine has recently undergone, new approaches, including that taken by proponents of the holistic health movement, have led to the frequent allocation of responsibility for illness to patients, their families, and occasionally to employers or the state.

In Japan, early socialization stresses individual and family responsibility for health and hygiene, and the occurrence of many types of illness is associated strongly with a sense of guilt and failure (DeVos and Wagatsuma 1959; Lebra 1982; Lock 1980). This is another reason for focusing on the somatic level in discussions about illness: it allows one to avoid dealing openly with the affect-laden psychological and social levels of explanation. The body is objectified, and discussion around it is dispassionate and incorporated into the world of *tatemae* and *soto,* although therapists, patients, and families are well aware of the implications of the discussion for the realms of *uchi* and *honne* (Long 1980).

This preliminary exploration should facilitate an interpretation of the data that follow on somatization and medicalization.[1]

The Vulnerable Female Body

The presentation of nonspecific complaints to a doctor in Japan is frequent and, as in North America, leads very often to overmedication, dissatisfaction among patients, and subsequent shopping around for other physicians. The expression for nonspecific complaints, *futeishūso,* is well known to everyone and, as in the West, is associated more frequently with women than with men. In a book entitled *Nonspecific Complaints: An Unknown Female Illness* (1980), three physicians working at a large Tokyo hospital tell the general public how they deal with this problem. They state that they have had thirty years' experience in this matter and have completely healed many women who had been suffering for years and were unable to get satisfactory medical help.

The problem of *futeishūso* is characterized by complaints about headaches, feelings of coldness *(hieshō),* shoulder stiffness (very common in Japan), dizziness, palpitations, nervousness, back pain, premenstrual pain, and feelings of depression, among many other symptoms. The three doctors believe these symptoms to be the result of something they call "chronic infectious pelvic disease" *(mansei kotsubannai kansenshō).* The existence of this disease, they add, cannot be proved at the present time, but they believe that it affects the autonomic nervous system, which, in turn, is the cause of the symptoms. They base their statements upon observation and treatment of five hundred patients who presented one or more of a total of fifty-six types of symptoms. The doctors claim that many women contract chronic infectious pelvic disease either as children or later in life; it occurs only in women because women's abdominal cavities are directly connected to the outside via the fallopian tubes, uterus, and vagina. When these tissues are damaged, particularly in association with miscarriages, abortions, childbirth, or ordinary menstruation, the way is open for bacterial infection. The doctors further state that the occurrence of an infection depends upon the "strength" of the bacteria and the resistance of the person in question; hence, physical responses vary greatly, but a mild chronic infection is very common.

The doctors have established diagnostic criteria for this disease that include symptoms of a malfunctioning autonomic nervous system, menstrual disorders, especially involving pain or the production of scarlet blood, and tenderness of the pelvic region. As treatment they recommend extended bed rest as well as avoidance of spicy foods, alcohol, overheating of the body, sexual intercourse, pregnancy, and most exercise. They recommend traditional herbal medicine as a preventive measure and professional consultation for anything more than a mild problem. Many of the patients of the authors of the book have been hospitalized, often for as long as fifty or sixty days. They are issued symptom charts that the women themselves check off each day; their diet is restricted, and the principal feature of their treatment is ice packs on the abdomen. When describing case histories, the authors take note of social and psychological dimensions, which they associate specifically with the onset of symptoms. Noted also is the transference experience of many patients, who talk openly for the first time in their lives with their doctors while undergoing the prolonged isolation in the hospital. But these aspects are not developed during or after leaving the hospital. Treatment is applied entirely at the physiological level, and the patients are returned to their former lives and situations.

The invention of this disease represents an interesting case of how biomedical "forms of medical treatment reinforce the perception that the 'truth' of human existence lies concealed within the confines of our own physical bodies" (Comaroff 1982, 59). The explanations given by the authors of *Nonspecific Complaints* possibly represent very careful observation and analysis of data; the book may be scientifically accurate up to a point, in that a bacillus may be a necessary factor in the onset of the illness. However, the numerous social and psychological reasons for differing human resistance to infection are not taken into consideration or dealt with to any extent, and the problem is treated in an extremely reductionistic fashion characteristic of much of biomedical practice.

The interchangeable terms *jiritsushinkeishūcho* (lack of harmony) or *jiritsusushinkeifuanteishō* (instability in the autonomic nervous system) are used very frequently by both Japanese physicians and patients. This categorization is often applied to cases that are hard to diagnose and that everyone readily agrees may have social or psychological implications. Both men and women can suffer from this problem, since it is agreed that "stressors" can affect the autonomic nervous system directly, but women tend to suffer from it more frequently. Explanations offered for the increased incidence among women vary. The most common is that, since hormonal changes influence the autonomic nervous system, women are prone to experience instability or lack of harmony in this system before menstruation or at menopause (which, in Japan, is usually considered to be a fifteen to twenty-year span). A second reason given for women's vulnerability is due to their disposition *(seishitsu),* which inclines them to be more nervous and hence easily stressed. A third interpretation given by a physician who is trained in traditional medicine as well as biomedicine is that "stale blood" *(oketsu)* collects in the female abdomen as the after result of childbirth and menstruation and affects the functioning of the autonomic nervous system.

Despite the apparent variations in interpretation described above, the focus of attention in each case is upon the physical body. Discussion centers around that apparently most scientific and abstract of terms "the autonomic nervous system" and the removal of unwanted symptoms, usually through hormones, tranquilizers, and sleeping pills.

Some informants, professional and otherwise, acknowledge that the use of "scientific" labels neutralizes the doctor-patient encounter, allowing it to proceed comfortably without incurring guilt or exposing the patient's private life too much. They also state that there really is not much that can be done about problems of the autonomic nervous system except to "stick it out"—*"gamman suru."* One "home doctor" book, put out by a small company known as the Life of the Housewife Press, after stating that no one knows if imbalance of the autonomic nervous system is really an illness or not and after giving a long list of symptoms, concludes that the best prevention is to review one's own habits and to try to improve them. Although clear assignment of guilt is avoided, responsibility for dealing with the problem is turned back to the patient and all discussion of social dynamics is studiously avoided (*Katei no igaku zenshu* 1983).

The Good Wife and Wise Mother

Two of the illnesses in modern Japan with the most striking names occur only to women: the "kitchen syndrome" and "moving-day depression." These ailments are not known by everyone, but the majority of the physicians interviewed had heard of the former and several of them the latter. The term "kitchen syndrome" was coined by Dr. Katsura Taisaku, who has had training in psychosomatic medicine and psychology and has written a book (1983) and several articles on the topic for the general public.

After ruling out serious organic malfunctioning, Dr. Katsura recommends the use of medication to control the symptoms but adds that the role of the physician is to listen and then to offer solutions by talking things over with the patient. All the physicians questioned on this subject agree that it is primarily a social problem, that Japanese women are still judged first and foremost by their roles as "good wife and wise mother" *(ryōsai kenbo),* and that, although they are well educated, there is virtually no possibility of their developing a sense of an independent identity *(jibun ga nai)* after they are married. Finding gainful employment other than in a factory is extremely difficult for a married women and is in any case socially frowned upon. The physicians also pointed out that women have no outlets for complaints. In the words of one specialist in internal medicine, "Many modern Japanese women are bored with their lives and they use 'organ language' to express this frustration, especially since the world of *tatemae* prohibits them from verbalizing their complaints."

In one case history documented by Dr. Katsura, the woman resorted to the use of men's linguistic forms; another patient went on wild shopping sprees; others suddenly started to buy food at random in addition to suffering from the kitchen syndrome. All these women had been people who formerly took great pride in their housework and in the organization of their family life.

Patients with moving-day depression also have numerous nonspecific complaints and are frequently diagnosed as depressed, although the rationalization for the symptoms by the patients themselves is often that the water in their new places of residence does not agree with them

(Sasaki 1983, 146). These patients, too, tend to be perfectionists who, after removal to a new part of Japan—almost without exception in connection with their husband's work—feel that their personalities have somehow changed and that they have become unable to run their homes as usual. Long rest and medication are advised for such cases. Frequently, husbands are noted as being sympathetic about their wives' illness, but this only serves to induce more guilt in the already sensitive women.

Recommendations by psychological oriented physicians for both of these problems are that some changes be made in the running of the household. It might be suggested, for example, that the family eat out now and again or that the mother not be expected to prepare several hot meals each evening as her children and husband return home one after the other. Taking up hobbies or a sport is also suggested, and occasionally it is recommended that the patient start some socially acceptable work (such as running a cookery school at home). Some of these recommendations no doubt help individual patients, sometimes very effectively, but the wider social ramifications of their problems are not held up for scrutiny. Although a physician might write a popular book on the subject of these ailments, thus offering the opportunity to question the social order, the issue is rarely taken up, and recommendations for treatment and change remain focused at the individual level.

Illnesses Caused by Mother

A well-established tradition in Japan holds mothers (and not parents) responsible for the health of their children, and *bogenbyō* (illnesses caused by the mother) are considered common occurrences. A well-known pediatrician, Dr. Kyūtoku Shigemori, has written a best-selling book (1979) and lectures widely on this subject. Dr. Kyūtoku believes there are two kinds of common colds, those caused by viruses and those originating in the upbringing of the child. Colds of the second type he classifies with childhood asthma and other psychosomatic problems as what he calls "diseases of civilization." He believes that although Japanese mothers were formerly good at child rearing, in the past twenty years they have become poor at it. Industrialization has distorted the "natural child-rearing instinct" into something that satisfies the mother's "narcissistic ego" but does not produce a healthy child. (The recorded incidence of asthma among children has doubled since the end of the war.) Mothers, Dr. Kyūtoku states, are usually too bossy or too protective. Another major problem is caused, he says, by the rise of the nuclear family, displacing the large, extended family, and the simultaneous urbanization of the nation. These developments isolate women, who cannot turn to the extended family for help and advice. Children who grow up in families such as this develop an unstable autonomic nervous system, the product of both genetics and environmental influences. Recommended treatment for severe cases is "parentectomy"—the removal of the child completely from the mother's charge for extended care in a hospital.

Dr. Kyūtoku believes that reduced breast feeding, overprotection of the child from climatic variation, and encouragement of passivity in the child are all factors contributing to childhood psychosomatic illnesses. While he thinks all children should be raised only by their own mothers until they are one year old, he acknowledges that this is not always a realistic possibility. Although he maintains that nursery schools were created not to raise the status of women but simply to exploit them as part of the labor force, he nevertheless adamantly opposes the widely held notion that mothers "abandon" *(suteru)* their children when they leave them in nursery schools. Dr. Kyūtoku stresses the view that mothers as much as children are victims of modern society and makes some practical suggestions for breaking down isolation and the sense of competition felt between Japanese mothers. He has recently written a book entitled *Fugenbyō* (Father-created illnesses), in which he attacks the organization of company work in Japan, which virtually precludes the involvement of fathers in the raising of their children.

Bogenbyō focuses largely on early socialization and child care and assumes the unproven existence of an inherent child-rearing instinct in women. The author, however, does raise the issue that analysis of the influence of modern Japanese society is crucial to finding lasting solutions to the majority of psychosomatic and somatic problems. At the same time, he retains a rather romantic notion of the extended family and the "good old days."

These examples serve to illustrate the various forms that medicalization can take in connection with nonspecific symptomatology and common psychosomatic problems. Some recommendations for change focus almost exclusively on the physical body, others incorporate both somatic treatment and suggestions for personal adjustment, while a few question, in addition, the social forces that contribute to oppression and resultant ill health. This variation is hardly surprising, given the complexity of Japanese society.

Images of Modern Middle-Class Japanese Women

Recent studies and government surveys of Japanese women (Kokumin Seikatsu Hakusho 1983; Lebra 1984a; Pharr 1976; White and Molony 1979) indicate that most middle-class women are largely satisfied with their roles as housewives and mothers and many of them enjoy their relatively easy life (although they do not usually see it as being easy) of housekeeping for a husband and family of two. Nevertheless, large numbers of women are bored, lonely, frustrated, and retain a strong feeling that they have no sense of personal identity or fulfillment. The rising divorce rate among fifty year olds is perhaps testimony to this situation (Madoka 1982). The following case studies illustrate some of these problems.

Mrs. Hori is a 49-year-old housewife whose oldest child is married; the second child has just entered college but lives at home. She is college educated, worked as a secretary until her marriage twenty years previously, and since that time has devoted her life to the care of her husband and children. Her husband works as the manager of a division of an electrical appliance firm that has branch offices throughout Japan. The Horis had been relocated once by the company when the children were young, and both of them had come to assume that they would not be moved again since this is less frequent in the case of senior managers. But Mr. Hori had been relocated three years earlier, at the age of fifty, to northern Kyushu, hundreds of miles from his home. The company assumed that Mrs. Hori and their younger child, who was still in high school at the time, would probably not accompany Mr. Hori and made no provisions for them to do so. Upon making extensive enquiries, it became clear to the Horis that no high school within a reasonable distance of the Kyushu branch office was prepared to take a new student. (There is no legal requirement that a child attend high school and therefore no obligation for a school to cooperate.) Mrs. Hori knew that even if they eventually were able to find a suitable school, her son would have difficulty in fitting in with a new group of students, and she had read several horrifying accounts to confirm her fears in this direction. Mrs. Hori foresaw that she, too, would have a problem fitting in. It is difficult to make meaningful new friendships in adult life in Japan, friends being almost exclusively composed of lifelong companions (Plath 1980, 161). Because her parents and closest friends would be seven hundred miles away, in Tokyo, Mrs. Hori could look forward to a life of isolation if she moved to Kyushu. She therefore decided very reluctantly to stay behind. Her friends and neighbors, many of them in a similar situation, told her that after a month or two she would get used to being without her husband; several of them added that, really, life is better without husbands anyway.

Mr. Hori had not been gone long before Mrs. Hori developed asthma and also started to suffer from frequent debilitating headaches. She talks of being bored and feeling sad and lonely much of the time, and adds that once her second son is married, her life will have no meaning. Shortly after her husband's departure Mrs. Hori started to take part in some local, slightly controversial political activity to relieve her boredom, but her husband was told by his company seniors to ask his wife to stop such activities because they might reflect badly upon the company. Mrs. Hori's doctor sympathizes with her situation, tells her that life is hard, and gives her medication for symptom relief. She expects nothing further from her doctor. Neither the Horis nor their family physician think that any alternative is possible to the present situation, although they all believe that Mrs. Hori's symptoms represent her distress about the family separation.

Mrs. Hori is ambivalent about her health problems. On the one hand, she feels somewhat embarrassed and guilty. She believes that she is not devoting herself fully to her son and that she causes other people trouble by being sick. On the other hand, she believes that she must endure this situation. She is resigned to it *(akiramete imasu),* and she has not tried the alternative traditional health care recommended by her neighbor. She does not seek to create a new life because she says that she was quite happy with the old one and, when pushed, admits that she has no confidence in her ability to do so. Since Mrs. Hori's husband is likely to be transferred back home from Kyushu in another few years, she is in an ambiguous position. Mrs. Hori's situation is a very common one in Japan, and for many women it may prove more difficult than divorce. The loss in such cases is seen as temporary, not a real loss, something to endure. Even though Mrs. Hori and those like her may have to endure for a considerable number of years, there are strong sanctions against creating anything new for themselves in compensation.

The practice of sending men away to work for extended periods, leaving behind wives and families, is not new; it is a tradition found among the samurai class in feudal Japan. Today it is widespread not only among businessmen (the Friday evening airplanes and long-distance trains are packed with men going home for the weekend) but also among farming families. The usual situation in the Japanese countryside today is for women to run the farm and raise the children while the men live in a neighboring town or city and work in an office or factory. The effects of an absent husband on all family members, not just wives, have yet to be investigated.

Several factors exacerbate the sense of loneliness and futility that many women feel. First, in a traditional family Mrs. Hori and others like her could expect, after working hard as "professional housewives" all their lives, to arrive, at the age of fifty, at the time of life when they would manage a large household but with a daughter-in-law doing most of the work. As a mother-in-law, the older Japanese woman in a traditional family enjoyed considerable power, freedom, and leisure. The nuclear family does not take away the mother-in-law's position, but it does convert it into a meaningless and empty privilege. The urban fifty year old today contemplates quite a different future from that of her predecessors. She lives in a small house with a husband who is often out for fourteen or fifteen hours a day. She and her husband usually expect to lead separate lives, and once the children are married a woman in a nuclear family is left with no sanctioned role except that of looking after her husband. Virtually no one will employ her, and she is expected to fill her day with hobbies of one kind or another. In fact, when asked what they do with their time, many women of this age reply that they sleep (see table 1). Vogel (1978) reports that older women often enjoy the freedom that a nuclear family offers and are happy not to be principally responsible for the grandchildren as was the case in an extended family, but other women complain that they can never "retire." A frequently used Japanese adage goes *"Teishu wa jōbu de rusu ga yoi"* (A good husband is one who is healthy and absent). In retirement many men may become excessively dependent upon their wives and insist that they always be present in the house to do the husband's slightest bidding (Vogel 1978, 35). Hence, subservience is all that many fifty-year-old women can look forward to in old age, a state that is compounded for many by caring for ailing and bedridden parents-in-law.

Of course, not everyone endures the situation stoically. Mrs. Morita, forty-five years old, is college educated, the mother of four children (unusual in modern Japan), and married to a man who works in an advertising company. The Moritas have not moved, and so Mrs. Morita does have some long-standing friends, including a group of women with whom she regularly meets and discusses her problems. Mr. Morita usually returns from work at ten o'clock every night of the week and expects a hot meal to be waiting for him. Mrs. Morita says that her husband complains about her all the time and has done so for years. He criticizes her appearance, the way she raises the children, and tells her that she does not sit or talk like a decent woman. Mrs. Morita also says that she has been hit "quite often" by her husband. She does not retaliate directly because she says she is afraid to do so, but she grumbles and weeps with her friends very readily. For the past five years whenever her husband has touched her, she has developed a florid skin rash at the point of contact; lately, even touching his dirty laundry has induced this response. The doctor whom Mrs. Morita occasionally consults has not suggested any form of help beyond medication. Mrs. Morita talks with her friends about a possible separation or divorce, but she believes, with considerable justification, that, given the Japanese legal system, she is likely to lose the children and/or to be left in a state of poverty and with no possible chance of employment.

Interviews with the wives of fifty-five businessmen confirm that the cases described above are not unusual (see table 1). These housewives, ranging in age between forty-five and fifty-five, live in nuclear families, with the exception of four whose in-laws reside with them. It must be stressed that although many women lead what to an outsider appears a rather dull life, thirty-eight out of the fifty-five respondents stated that

Table 1. **Daily Routine of Housewives**

	%	N=55
Three hours or less spent in housework per day, on average	89	49
Full-time work	0	0
Part-time work, 1–4 hours per day	16	9
Involvement in community activities once a week or more	20	11
Weekly involvement in hobbies or recreation outside of home	56	31
Three or more hours spent actively watching TV per day	51	28
Reading for one hour or more each day	5	3
One hour or less spent with husband each weekday	80	44
A daytime nap taken most days	27	15
Visits from or to friends, weekly or more	22	12

they were happy with their lives. Of the seventeen who were not happy, twelve attributed it to their very poor marital relationship, and two added that their children were not doing well, which compounded their unhappiness. Ten said that the lack of companionship was their major problem. All of the respondents expressed the belief that their unhappiness affects their health, and eighteen of them complained of recurring physical symptoms of various kinds. Of the total sample of fifty-five, fifty-three respondents believe that a woman is largely responsible for her own health and illness, although it is agreed that infections and serious diseases cannot usually be avoided. When asked what changes might improve their lives, ten of the fifty-five respondents said that they were thinking about trying to find a part-time job; five of those added that their husbands are against such an idea. The other forty-five had no ideas of any kind for improving their lives and added that they were tired of PTA work, housework, and consumer groups and often dissatisfied with their recreational activities as well.

Clearly, one cannot make any accurate generalizations from this small sample, but the results suggest a number of variables that should be investigated with a larger group of respondents. These include class differences and differences between women living in extended and nuclear families, living with and without supportive husbands, with and without children at home, as well as differences between women who have and have not moved and those who do and do not work. These variables need to be compared and then correlated with the occurrence of symptoms, physician visits, the use of medication, and the use of support groups.[2]

Conclusion

Modern Japanese society is perceived as very stressful by those who participate in it. There is one group of people, middle-class housewives, who are often singled out as an exception. Housewives are thought in general to enjoy an easy and rather spoilt life-style. Their daily round is sarcastically characterized as *san shoku hiru ne tsuki* (a permanent job with three meals and a nap thrown in). Many women enjoy the role of *sengyō shufu* (professional housewife), and make the most of the leisure time associated with that role. Others, however, fret over their lack of self-identity, and a considerable number suffer unremitting feelings of loneliness and oppression. Those who suffer believe themselves to be stressed and can usually articulate what they perceive to be the nub of their problem: discordant family relations, sometimes exacerbated by physical separation, and an inability on their part to endure the situation. If physical symptoms occur, the woman and her family are likely to interpret them as a response to stress. There is an ongoing dialectic between stress and symptomatology, in which either variable, depending upon the particular context, can be considered as causal of the other, and in which intervening psychological states do not usually figure to any great extent. The occurrence of sickness in women is not altogether acceptable in Japan. Males can be dependent, but women must nurture and nourish the family, and guilt associated with illness is particularly acute for women, who often believe that their whole family will suffer in turn (Lock 1982). However, if symptoms can be legitimized through a doctor's opinion or by appropriate labeling (see Rosenberger, this volume), then somatization becomes a powerful form of nonconfrontational communication. Women themselves, therefore, tend to welcome medicalization of their problems; many of them actively seek out professional care and willingly imbibe medication for problems that they believe originate in social conflict.

Features of Japanese social organization that disparage open confrontation, and encourage nonverbal communication and self-responsibility for health and illness, function to focus the attention of both physicians and patients upon the physical body and appropriate somatically oriented therapies. The reductionistic thinking characteristic of biomedicine coupled with a strong reliance on technology add to this tendency, which is further exacerbated by a largely unquestioned business ethic in medicine. Physicians derive much of their income from the sale of medication, and many of them also run private clinics for profit. There is considerable incentive for Japanese physicians to try to exert control over a population of people in distress (although this is somewhat countered by the fact that the majority of people are cared for by a general practitioner with whom they have a close, lifelong relationship [see Steslicke and Long, this volume]). Excessive use is made of medication in Japan (Sakuma 1969) but not simply, I think, as a result of physicians acting in their own interest. It is also due to an aggressive pharmaceutical industry and can, in part, be attributed to a willing and gullible public.

Medication and the small life-style modifications suggested by professionals for some women no doubt often help to ease the sense of oppression that patients experience. At the same time, medicalization can act as an "opiate," and can deflect attention away from the social origins of distress. Lebra (1984b) warns about some of the problems that can arise when nonconfrontational modes of dealing with conflict are widely used; quiet or subtle messages can easily be ignored. Moreover, the sufferer's easy access to medication can facilitate avoidance of receiving the message directed at the offender, whether it be a husband, an employer, or the state.

Women often link their allergies, asthmas, stiff shoulders, and poorly functioning autonomic nervous systems to their immediate social relationships, and especially to their subordination to their husbands and other people who figure centrally in their lives. They may sometimes tentatively question these relationships, but they rarely see the links between the structure of society at large and female subordination in general (Cook and Hayashi 1980). Nor do they seriously question the pressures imposed by the larger, fiercely competitive society on all its members. Female protest about the stress they experience is usually expressed through their own bodies and by griping and gossiping about their immediate family members. There are exceptions to this, and some women's groups have organized to promote change, but they are relatively rare.

In the actual clinical encounter, the social origins of distress are not explored to any great extent; nevertheless, the titles of the books that medical professionals are currently producing indicate that they are aware of at least some of the social ramifications of their patients' problems. Like many of the women themselves, the majority of health professionals writing popular books hold a rather negative stereotype of women. Women's general physical vulnerability to sickness is widely accepted; prevalent also is the belief that, unlike women of previous generations, women today lack self-control and the ability to suppress individual needs. Moreover, a life of ease dominated by extravagant and selfish motives made possible through the rise of the nuclear family and rapid economic development is considered central in the undoing of the "good wife and wise mother" (Lock 1986). The authors of many of these books sermonize about weak and willful women and suggest several ways in which they should "shape up." However, in delivering their harangue, the books' authors inadvertently reveal chronic points of stress and tension in Japanese society, usually associated with the subordinate position of women (despite their official equality [Pharr 1984]) in the family and the workplace. They also sometimes reveal the way that business and the state exploit individuals and families by the expectation that personal needs be subordinated almost without exception to the demands of business and industry. Popular literature on the subject mercilessly depicts the life of the "salary man," for example, as mindless, pointless, and totally exploited by his employers (Skinner 1979).

In societies where social participation in ritual events is commonplace, there is the opportunity for women to readily discover that their distress is shared by others (Comaroff 1985; Parsons 1984), and articulation of social problems can then be facilitated through collective ritual performance. The alienation of middle-class urban dwellers is increased by isolation, and there is no opportunity to understand how common their problems are nor to appreciate their social rather than personal origins. The popular literature written by physicians is not uniform, it gives a range of opinions, and some of it, such as the book by Kyūtoku, raises for scrutiny a few of the paradoxes and contradictions in the lives of modern Japanese women and their families, thereby allowing an attentive reader to become sensitive to alternative possibilities. Certainly the writing of popular books lines the pockets of physicians, just as it functions to medicalize a problem (since none of the physicians disassociate themselves from giving care). But if at the same time some of this literature acts as a catalyst in breaking down the isolation and oppression of middle-class women, then it might also sow the seeds for future de-medicalization of that problem and pave the way for some appropriation of control by the women involved.

Notes

1. Data presented in this study are the results of work in progress and have been obtained from textual sources and open-ended interviews with twelve physicians (internists and gynecologists) and fifty-five urban middle-class housewives.

2. This research is at present in progress with a sample of 1,700 women.

References

Akaeda, H., K. Akaeda, and O. Akaeda. 1980. *Shirarezaru fujin byō* (Nonspecific female complaints). Tokyo: Fujin Seikatsu Sha.

Bellah, R. 1957. *Tokugawa religion*. Glencoe, Ill.: Free Press.

———. 1962. Values and social change in modern Japan. *Asian Cultural Stud-*

ies. Reprinted in R. Bellah. 1970. *Beyond belief.* New York: Harper and Row.

Comaroff, J. 1982. Medicine. In *The problem of medical knowledge,* ed. A. Treacher and P. Wright. Edinburgh: Edinburgh Univ. Press.

———. 1985. *Body of power, spirit of resistance.* Chicago: Univ. of Chicago Press.

Cook, A. H., and H. Hayashi. 1980. *Working women in Japan.* Cornell International Industrial and Labor Relations Report No. 10. Ithaca.

Devisch, R. 1985. Symbol and psychosomatic symptom in bodily space-time. *International Journal of Psychology* 20:396–412.

DeVos, G. 1973. Socialization for achievement. Berkeley and Los Angeles: Univ. of California Press.

DeVos, G., and H. Wagatsuma. 1959. Psychocultural significance of concern over death and illness among rural Japanese. *International Journal of Social Psychiatry* 5:5–19.

Doi, T. 1973. *The anatomy of dependence.* Tokyo: Kodansha.

Ehrenreich, J. 1978. *The cultural crisis of modern medicine.* New York: Monthly Review Press.

Frankenberg, R. 1980. Medical anthropology and development. *Social Science and Medicine* 14B:197–207.

Freidson, E. 1970. *Profession of medicine.* New York: Dodd, Mead and Co.

Gaines, A. D., and R. A. Hahn. 1985. *Physicians of western society.* Boston: D. Reidel.

Good, B. 1977. The heart of what's the matter. *Culture, Medicine and Psychiatry* 1:25–28.

Guttmacher, S. 1979. Whole in body, mind and spirit. *Hastings Center Report,* April.

Gramsci, A. 1971. *Selections from the prison notebooks.* New York: International Publishers.

Habermas, J. 1971. *Towards a rational society.* London: Heinemann.

Harootunian, H. D. 1974. Between politics and culture. In *Japan in crisis,* ed. H. D. Harootunian and B. S. Silberman. Princeton: Princeton Univ. Press.

Helman, C. 1985. Psyche, soma, and society. *Culture, Medicine and Psychiatry* 9:1–26.

Illich, I. D. 1976. *Medical nemesis.* New York: Pantheon.

Kamishima, J. 1973. *Nihon kindaika no tokushitsu* (Special features of Japanese modernization). Tokyo: Ajia Keizai Kenkyūjo.

Katei no igaku zenshū (Collected writings on household medicine). 1983. Tokyo: Kabushiki Kaisha Fujia Seikatsu Shashuppanbu.

Katsura, T. 1983. *Daidokoro shōkōgun* (The kitchen syndrome). Tokyo: Sanmaku Shuppan.

Kleinman, A. 1979. *Patients and healers in the context of culture.* Berkeley and Los Angeles: Univ. of California Press.

———. 1982. Neurasthenia and depression. *Culture, Medicine and Psychiatry* 6:117–190.

Kokumin Seikatsu Hakusho. 1983. *Keizai kikakuchō* (Signs in economic planning). Tokyo: Ōkura Insatsu Kyoku.

Koschmann, V. 1978. *Authority and the individual in Japan.* Tokyo: Univ. of Tokyo Press.

Krause, E. A. 1977. *Power and illness.* New York: Elsevier.

Krauss, E. S. 1974. *Japanese radicals revisited.* Berkeley and Los Angeles: Univ. of California Press.

Krauss, E. S., T. P. Rohlen, and P. G. Steinhoff. 1984. *Conflict in Japan.* Honolulu: Univ. of Hawaii Press.

Kyūtoku, S. 1979. *Bogenbyō* (Illnesses caused by Mother). Tokyo: Sanmaku Shuppan.

Lebra, T. 1974. Interactional perspective on suffering and curing in a Japanese cult. *International Journal of Social Psychiatry* 20:281–286.

———. 1976. *Japanese patterns of behavior.* Honolulu: Univ. of Hawaii Press.

———. 1982. Self-reconstruction of faith healing. In *Cultural conceptions of mental health and therapy,* ed. A. J. Marsella and G. M. White. Boston: D. Reidel.

———. 1984a. *Japanese women.* Honolulu: Univ. of Hawaii Press.

———. 1984b. Nonconfrontational strategies for management of interpersonal conflicts. In *Conflict in Japan,* ed. E. S. Krauss, T. P. Rohlen, and P. G. Steinhoff. Honolulu: Univ. of Hawaii Press.

Lewis, I. M. 1971. *Ecstatic religion.* Middlesex: Penguin.

Lock, M. 1980. *East Asian medicine in urban Japan.* Berkeley and Los Angeles: Univ. of California Press.

———. 1982. Traditional and popular attitudes towards mental health and illness in Japan. In *Cultural conceptions of mental health and therapy,* ed. A. J. Marsella and G. M. White. Boston: D. Reidel.

———. 1986. Plea for acceptance. *Social Science and Medicine* 23:99–112.

Long, S. O. 1980. Fame, fortune, and friends. Ph.D. diss. University of Illinois, Urbana.

MacPherson, K. I. 1981. Menopause as disease. *Advances in Nursing Science* 3:95–113.

Madoka, Y. 1982. *Shufushōkōgun* (The housewife syndrome). Tokyo: Bunda Shuppankyoku.

Mechanic, D. 1980. The experience and reporting of common physical complaints. *Journal of Health and Social Behavior* 21:146–155.

Merkin, D. H. 1976. *Pregnancy as a disease.* Port Washington, New York: Kennikat Press.

Minuchin, S., L. Baker, and B. L. Rosman. 1978. *Psychosomatic families.* Cambridge: Harvard Univ. Press.

Murray, P. 1975. The idioms of contemporary Japan, 12. *The Japan Interpreter* 10:90–95.

Nichter, M. 1981. Idioms of distress. *Culture, Medicine and Psychiatry* 5:379–408.

Parsons, C. D. F. 1984. Idioms of distress. *Culture, Medicine and Psychiatry* 8:71–93.

Pharr, S. J. 1976. The Japanese woman. In *Japan, the paradox of progress,* ed. L. Austen. New Haven: Yale Univ. Press.

———. 1984. Status conflict. In *Conflict in Japan,* ed. E. S. Krauss, T. P. Rohlen, and P. G. Steinhoff. Honolulu: Univ. of Hawaii Press.

Plath, D. W. 1980. Long engagements. Stanford: Stanford Univ. Press.

Reynolds, D. K. 1976. *Morita psychotherapy.* Berkeley and Los Angeles: Univ. of California Press.

———. 1980. *The quiet therapies.* Honolulu: Univ. of Hawaii Press.

Sakuma, A. 1969. *Kusuri to karada* (Medication and the body). Tokyo: Tokyo Univ. Press.

Sasaki, H. 1983. *Kokoro no kenkō sōdanshitsu* (Consultations for mental health). Tokyo: Asahi Shimbunsha.

Simmel, G. 1969. *Conflict and the web of group affiliations.* New York: Free Press.

Skinner, K. 1979. Sarariiman manga (Comic strips about salary men). *The Japan Interpreter* 12 (3–4): 449–457.

Stark, E. 1982. Doctors in spite of themselves. *International Journal of Health Services* 12:419–457.

Szasz, T. 1970. *The manufacture of madness.* New York: Harper and Row.

Tsurumi, K. 1972. *Kōkishin to nihonjin* (Curiosity and the Japanese). Tokyo: Kodansha.

———. 1974. Shakai to henka no atarashii paradaimu (New paradigms for society and social change). In *Shisō no bōken* (Adventures in thought), ed. S. Ichii and K. Tsurumi. Tokyo: Tsukuma Shobō.

Vogel, S. 1978. Professional housewife. *The Japan Interpreter* 12:16–43.

Waitzkin, H., and B. Waterman. 1974. *The exploitation of illness in capitalist society.* Indianapolis: Bobbs-Merrill.

White, J. W. 1984. Protest and change in contemporary Japan. In *Institutions for change in Japanese society,* ed. G. DeVos. Berkeley: Institute of East Asian Studies, Univ. of California Press.

White, M. I., and B. Moloney, eds. 1979. Proceedings of the Tokyo symposium on women. Tokyo: International Group for the Study of Women.

Yoshida, T. 1984. Spirit possession and village conflict. In *Conflict in Japan,* ed. E. S. Krauss, T. P. Rohlen, and P. G. Steinhoff. Honolulu: Univ. of Hawaii Press.

Young, A. 1976. Internalizing and externalizing medical belief systems. *Social Science and Medicine* 10:147–156.

———. 1982. Anthropology of sickness. *Annual Review of Anthropology* 11:257–285.

Zola, I. K. 1978. Medicine as an institution of social control. In *The cultural crisis of modern medicine,* ed. J. Ehrenreich. New York: Monthly Review Press.

Productivity, Sexuality, and Ideologies of Menopausal Problems in Japan

NANCY R. ROSENBERGER

Japan has been presented in much of the literature as a homogenous society in which there is little variety or conflict. This homogeneity is said to have been reinforced in recent years by the widespread use of television, radio, and newspapers, and the commonality of education materials. I believe that there is, in fact, variety and conflict within Japanese society. In this chapter, I discuss some of the variation in values that exists among middle-aged women and examine differences in their households and in their ideas and actions concerning menopausal symptoms.

My contention is that in Japan many ideas and actions related to the menopause vary in response to middle-aged women's current problems with the household and their position in it. Thus, middle-aged women use ideas and actions around menopausal symptoms as one way of manipulating their place (or lack of it) as productive people within the society, especially within the household.

Productivity is important to the Japanese, important in the sense that every person is expected, if possible, to be a participating member of a group (Smith 1983; Lebra 1976; Nakane 1970). It is not required that the person's contribution achieve high levels of productivity in an industrial sense, but it is important that a Japanese person show the right attitude of support and participation in the group of main membership. Passive members of groups are accepted if those people are considered too young, too old, or in some way infirm. However, middle-aged women are not ordinarily granted the role of passive participant by themselves or others. Productivity is expected, but problems stem from how that productivity is expressed in various social contexts in contemporary Japan.

The assumption that ideas and actions in connection with menopause have some inherent relation to problems of productive group membership in Japan rests on the definition of the female gender primarily in social terms. Although there are individual interpretations and variations, several commonly held ideas about women underlie the definition of a woman as a socially understood gender. "Woman" in Japan is defined first and foremost by her sexuality, which implies reproductive capabilities (manifested through menstruation), by reproduction of children, by reproduction of household members, by productive membership in her husband's household, and by personality traits of gentleness, nurturance, and self-control (Rosenberger 1984b). The latter traits are thought to develop in their most ideal form through a woman's experience within a household—through raising children, nurturing a husband, and caring for parents-in-law. To the extent that she has done these things, a woman is regarded as mature in a womanly fashion.

The menopause marks a departure from sexuality (defined by menstruation) and the capability of reproduction. If the woman has reproduced in her husband's household, she maintains her womanly role as a mother (and perhaps mother-in-law), as a productive member of the household, and through her personality traits. Lebra states that Japanese women "never graduate from the maternal role" (1984, 260), but active service in relation to this role does decrease when children leave. If children have left the household, temporarily or permanently, it is the woman's productive membership within the household that is left as the most convenient way of expressing her gender in "traditional" social terms. In addition, the woman may work outside the home, usually to make an economic contribution to household needs and in part for her own self-interest. It will be seen in the third part of this essay that Tokyo women show an increasing interest in productivity outside the household and are interpreting this as part of their personhood, quite in tune with their definition of contemporary gender roles.

In short, I am positing that as other qualities that define the female gender in social terms disappear in middle age, Japanese women tend to find their productive membership in the household or in society to be important. Menopausal symptoms in no way determine the form of productivity that the woman finds meaningful to express herself as a productive female person. However, a woman manipulates the ideas and actions that are attached to menopause to explain to herself and others the forms of productivity that she has chosen. Thus, the place of the

household in the economy, the woman's forms of productive membership within the household, and other areas of productivity available to
her outside the household are important to understanding the various
ways in which she will use (or refuse to use) menopausal symptoms to
express herself in a way that is commensurate with her expected social
roles. When viewed in this manner, it can be understood why menopausal symptoms, while not considered to be important to middle-aged
women as a biological transition, can have importance on the social level.

A similar relationship between menopause and productive membership may occur in other societies in which, like Japan, there is no special
ritual or public role for women after menopause. Women in such
societies do not necessarily use ideas or actions about menopause as a
means of dealing with their problems of social gender in middle age, but
ideas and action around menopause are a potential way for middle-aged
women to label and handle problems in connection with a definition of
themselves as productive female persons in their households or in the
larger society.

Many studies have explored the relationship of status to the menopausal experience; several researchers (Bart 1969; Flint 1979; Moaz et al.
1970; Brown 1982) have argued that the reporting of menopausal symptoms is high in places where women's status is low, whereas menopausal
symptoms are fewer and less often reported in places where women's status is high after menopause. Davis (1982) found that for her Newfoundland informants, high status is lifelong and does not change at menopause, and that people worry about the menopause and use it to
emphasize the importance of their role, their hard work, and their stoic
nature.

I have attempted in the following discussion to avoid generalization
about the correlation of status and menopausal symptoms. However, my
thesis is that Japanese women use the images connected with the menopausal sufferer in order to enhance their personal status as productive
female persons, regardless of their actual status in the view of the larger
society.

Neither am I concerned to show here which symptoms are identified
with the menopause in Japan (see Lock 1986), nor what physical factors
might be influencing menopausal symptoms (Beyene 1984). My interest
is with whether symptoms experienced in middle age are emphasized by
women in certain contexts, whether these middle-aged symptoms are
identified as menopausal, and what this identification (or lack of it) can

explain. The concern is with menopause as part of an ideology, if you will, that is used by women to adjust to or to manipulate (both ·consciously and unconsciously) their place in the social and economic specificities of their lives as middle-aged women. In more general terms, this study examines how health and illness states connected with natural bodily transitions are used by the people identified with them to control or manipulate their positions in the socioeconomic situations in which they find themselves.

Despite the attempt to avoid a static analysis by discussing variety and conflict, even the three contexts presented below become three fixed models in the act of recording them. In each of the areas discussed women actually have many individual approaches to the menopause and its usefulness (or lack thereof) in relation to the problems of middle life. The generalities presented below are the dominant patterns that have emerged from the particular data of this researcher. Women's ideas and actions regarding their productive membership in middle age (especially within the household) and the use of the menopause in relation to that productive membership is constantly in flux, even within the daily life of one woman. For example, in a group of well-educated working women, a woman may use menopause to define her position as a working person by denying any menopausal symptoms. The same woman, in a group of chatting neighbors on the street outside her home, may use menopausal symptoms to emphasize her dissatisfactions at home. In short, the reader is asked to bear in mind that the ideas presented here are frozen patterns in a process that is continually in flux in each locality and, indeed, for each person.

The term "household" is used here in a historically specific sense. In its so-called traditional form, the household in Japan was an economic, political, and ritual entity that had at its core a line of co-head married pairs, ideally related through a line of elder sons (Bachnik 1983; Brown 1966; Kitaoji 1971). Daughters could carry on the household if their husbands married into their line, but women never created new households without bringing in a husband. As Bachnik (1983) has noted, the continuation of the household as an entity rather than the continuation of the line was most important.

I base my use of the term "household" on the above definition, which ideologically is still the ideal of the household in Japan. The household in contemporary Japan seldom rests on economic and political functions, but rather on its ideological or ritual functions (Brown 1966). The ideal of the household as an ongoing line of elder sons, co-residential or close in proximity, is still the cherished ideal of middle-aged women in the northeastern provincial city studied. It is questionable to what extent the household as an ideological entity is important for the Tokyo women who are presented in the study. From the point of view of many female informants living in Tokyo, the care of the individual members of the nuclear family is of greater concern than is the ongoing idea of the household. The reader is cautioned that in Tokyo, and to a lesser extent in the provincial city, co-residence of the continuing line is greatly reduced and care is offered increasingly on the basis of emotional attachment and kindred rather than on the basis of the household. Nevertheless, the ideal of the woman's actions within the "traditional" household is the source of the definition of the woman's appropriate actions in relation to her family members (of all generations) even among the well educated of Tokyo. In addition, Japanese women's identities become increasingly linked with the continuation of the household as they age (Lebra 1984). For these reasons, the term "household" is used throughout this paper to express the framework in which actions of family-oriented productivity are accomplished.

The data on which this analysis rests were collected in Japan between 1980 and 1983. The first area of research was in a provincial city in Iwate prefecture, a prefecture in northeastern Honshu characterized as being "traditional" in customs and comparatively backward economically. My data were collected in two ways: in-depth interviews and questionnaires. Sixty women were interviewed in their homes or in a doctor's office; 189 women responded to a questionnaire on menopause and other aspects of their life such as work and home relations. The second part of the research was done in Tokyo, where I interviewed 100 women who were coming into the hospital for a routine yearly checkup. They were healthy women who were interviewed about various aspects of their lives—their hobbies, work, family relations, as well as ideas and actions related to menopause—and responded to a questionnaire on attitudes toward menopause. The last part of the research was done in a small fishing-farming village in Iwate prefecture where 30 women were interviewed. These interviews mostly took place in the women's homes; a few were conducted in a community center when being in the home would have constrained the conversation. Doctors in each of these research locations were interviewed on their views of menopause, the associated symptoms, causes, and cures.

The majority of women interviewed were in "middle age" (defined for the purpose of this study as forty to sixty years of age). A lesser number of women in their thirties and sixties were interviewed for comparison. The ages forty to sixty seem appropriate for the Japanese case because by the time most women are forty all of their children are in school (thirty-five is usually considered by Japanese women to be the cutoff age for giving birth), and by sixty, most women are grandmothers, their husbands are completely retired, and the effects of menopause are supposed to be finished. The age from sixty to seventy is sometimes referred to as "early old age." Where "menopausal" is used as a label for middle-aged symptoms, the time period from forty to sixty is considered to be an appropriate age range for menopausal symptoms to appear. Thus, the term "menopausal" as it is used in parts of Japan includes long periods prior to and after cessation of menstruation in which the body is thought to be susceptible to the effects of changing hormones.

The Path of Blood

The first set of ideas and actions in relation to menopause is that conveyed to the researcher by the women of the fishing-farming village in northeastern Japan. Even by rural Japanese standards, this village is somewhat unique in that it had been cut off from other towns except by foot or boat until approximately ten years prior to the interviews. Up to that point, most households in this village were responsible for their own subsistence, providing themselves with vegetables, soy sauce, miso, fish, rice, and so on. Trading for fish and rice went on between those households that concentrated on fishing or farming, but many households both farmed and fished. The woman of the household was responsible for the growing and preservation of vegetables and the making of staples such as tofu, miso, and soy sauce. She helped prepare the fish that her husband brought in either to sell or for household consumption and helped with the rice (planting, weeding, and harvesting) to an extent determined by the husband's involvement in fishing or charcoal making. In short, the economic role of the woman in the household was quite important and continued to be so as long as she was able to contribute.

The custom, among common folk since at least the Meiji period, of having the eldest son (eldest daughter if no son) and his family live with and carry on the household is still considered to be vital and is usually maintained in this village today. Thus, middle-aged women are busy supplying food for their growing families and helping to care for grand-children. Middle-aged women have often given birth in their forties and usually have four to six children rather than the prescribed two found in most of Japan. There are thus both younger children who have not yet left home and grandchildren living together in most village households. The woman's roles as mother and grandmother therefore overlap, and her productive role in the household is never interrupted. As the middle-aged woman inherits the role of mother-in-law in directing the affairs of the household and makes use of the labor of her daughter-in-law, her power is increased.

The ideas and actions of these women toward menopause are classed here under the phrase *"chi no michi,"* literally, "path of blood." This phrase originates in traditional medicine, where it refers to all womanly problems that have any connection with childbearing or menstruation. It is still used by village women over about fifty years of age, usually with reference to health problems thought to be associated with the female reproductive organs or cycle, and is understood by all. Its meaning describes well these women's ideas about menopause. Colloquially, the "path of blood" represents the idea that menopausal distress results from passing through the functions unique to the female (menstruation, births, and menopause). As one informant said:

> We women spend our whole lives being "threatened by blood" *(chi ni odakasareru).* I used to look at my mother suffering through meno-pause and think I'd never be like her. But here I am. It's a path no woman can avoid.

The most threatening time along the "path of blood" is thought to be the postbirth period. It was described graphically by one informant:

> It wasn't like now when the nurses massage your uterus to get the blood out. After the baby was born, blood sometimes got left in there and got rotten like. It stays in there and causes problems later on in the menopausal years.

The appeal of the "path of blood" lies in the fact that the aches and pains attributed to menopause are associated by inference with the whole path of a woman's reproductive life. Thus, discussion of aches attributed to the "path of blood" refers the listener back to the hard work and effort put into pregnancies, childbirths, and childrearing in the context of the household. In this case, menopause is not a stage of life in which children are gone and the woman is alone in the household; rather menopausal symptoms are interpreted as the product of years of hard work as the mother in a household and are linked with the need for help with that hard work in the future. Menopausal symptoms interpreted as the "path of blood" emphasize the village woman's position in the household and her continuing sacrifice for the household upon which her authority depends.

In the following two conversations, we meet one village woman who claims she did have menopausal problems and another who claims she did not. In both cases the idea being stressed by the informant is her hard work and devotion within her household.

Mrs. Okuchi, the elder wife in a household including herself, her husband, her eldest son, his wife, and four grandchildren, dominated the conversation as her husband and daughter-in-law sat quietly in the circle around the wood-burning stove.

It's those women in the cities who are rich with nothing to do who get menopausal problems. Women who work outside of the home get menopausal symptoms—like my daughter-in-law here. You know, young people want a lot of material comforts. If you get out in the fields and move your body, women don't have much trouble with the path of blood.

(Did you have much difficulty around menopause?)

Well, I did. My period ended soon after the birth of my seventh child. He was born when I was forty, and I got very sick the summer I was forty-two. I had a fever and was down in bed for three months.

(Why would your menopause have been so difficult?)

I guess it was because I worked so hard and had so many babies. We were poor and I could never rest after the births, except for the first one. I just kept going. There was no one else to tend the vegetables because my husband was off taking care of the charcoal making in the mountains, and most of my family had died in the tidal wave.

Ten years after my last child, my son's first child was born, so I was busy being a grandmother. No, around here we can't stop to worry about the path of blood.

Mrs. Okuchi's original emphasis on the idea that people who work in the fields do not get menopausal problems can be understood through the high value that is placed on endurance without complaint and continual productivity for women of this village. When brought up in a general context, menopausal aches are treated with disdain because they represent the idea that a woman gives in to her individual problems, thus ignoring the needs of the family group. However, when admitted to on a personal level, as above, menopausal problems are immediately associated with the sacrifices that the woman has made for the household and the family. In either situation (denying or admitting to menopausal symptoms), the woman's response emphasizes the fulfillment of her duty as central household worker and mother.

Mrs. Muto is fifty-eight and runs a small inn with the help of her daughter-in-law. We talked over tea in her parlor.

> Some women get the path of blood, but not me. I just didn't think about it. Some have it even in their late thirties, but I had none. I was too busy working and I had to keep going. Until five years ago, I had to walk several miles and carry our store-bought supplies on my back. Until just recently, we grew all of the vegetables we ate. I was responsible for that because my husband was off on a boat for six months a year to New Zealand. I still make our bean curd and soy sauce. I have no time for the path of blood.

In short, women of this fishing-farming village preferred to portray themselves as immune to menopausal problems and emphasized instead their domestic and reproductive labor for the household. If they did admit to problems that they thought had been connected with the menopause, it was done in the framework of the "path of blood," the natural way of things for a woman who had given so much for her household.

These ideas around menopause are best understood through the economic vitality of the household in village subsistence and the centrality of the woman to household production. The definition of women as socially accepted females and as productive people stems simultaneously from their reproductive and domestic labor within the household. Women's explanations of menopausal symptoms and their preference for denying menopausal symptoms can be traced to their central roles in households with continuing economic and social importance.

Village women in their late twenties and early thirties added an interesting perspective to the way their mothers-in-law dealt with menopausal symptoms. They agreed that women of the older generation were strong both in body and spirit, so that they could put up with whatever aches they had. They added, however, that their mothers-in-law were quite loquacious about their menopausal problems when they wanted to convince a household member to do something for them or to act in a certain manner. Thus, if her menopausal symptoms could help to motivate a child to do well in a test for "your sick grandmother who's taken care of you and your papa," the grandmother would reveal her menopausal problems without shame or embarrassment. In one case the mother-in-law's menopausal symptoms were the deciding factor in convincing the elder son and his wife to move into the main house from the smaller house next door. Using sickness as a means of motivating action in others is not new in the literature about Japan (see Caudill 1962; Ohnuki-Tierney 1984). These particular uses of menopause fit well into the idea that menopause can be used in this village to bring the middle-aged woman into an ever more emotional and obligatory relationship with the members of her household at a time when her declining reproductive and sexual powers could threaten her status within the household.

Problems of the Menopausal Years

In the provincial city, menopausal distress is referred to as *kōnenki shō-gai*, "problems of the menopausal years." While the "path of blood" carries the idea that female suffering occurs along a continuum, the phrase "problems of the menopausal years" carries the idea that menopausal distress happens within a confined period of time. The *nenki* of *kōnenki* means "period of time" or "stage." The *kō* carries several meanings: it has the meaning of "again" and in combination with other characters conveys the idea of change. *Kō* also refers to the time from sunset to sunrise, divided into segments as for the night watch; accordingly, it is used in verb form to mean "growing late" *(fukeru)* or in combination, "getting deep into the night" *(fukeyuku)*. Thus, *kōnenki* could be translated as the "darkening years," with the image of the woman progressing into night at menopause. The image of night complements the image of the sun used to represent menstruation in young women in Japan.[1]

Shōgai, the second part of the phrase used to mean "menopausal problems," is used in the medical world to refer to certain kinds of damage or disability, but it can also mean "hurdles," as in a horse race. Although this is not the meaning that biomedical doctors intend, it is not irrelevant to the ideas surrounding "problems of the menopausal years." When Japanese talk of passing through this period, they say that a woman has to "ride over" *(norikoeru)* the "problems of the meno-pausal years." A doctor writes about "menopausal problems" in a popu-lar health magazine:

> For a woman, the end of menses must be shocking. Her functions as a woman are ended and she leaves her youth, beauty and feminine attractiveness behind . . . the decline of her body is rapid with loosening of skin . . . decline of sex life . . . and weakening of memory . . . In the home she is freed from child care, but she tastes the feelings of loneliness and loss of her role as mother. She can no longer get fulfillment from her household duties. Besides that, she worries about her husband's retirement and his relations with other women. (Kawashima 1978, 230–231)

"The menopausal years" *(kōnenki)* demarcates a period between the years of "maturity" or "young motherhood" *(seijukuki)* and the "years of old age" *(rōnenki)*. Most contemporary Japanese women do not pro-ceed from motherhood into grandmotherhood as Mrs. Okuchi of the fishing village did, with only ten years between her last child and her first grandchild. The usual gap between children and grandchildren today is between twenty and thirty years, as the average number of chil-dren has decreased and children marry later than did the present middle-aged generation.[2] The grandparent is likely to live separately from her grandchildren until she needs care herself. The average age of meno-pause in Japan is estimated to be ten years later than it was at the end of World War II, so that in 1979 the average age of menopause was fifty-two years of age.[3] Thus, for fifteen to twenty years before menopause, the woman is rarely busy with child care. It is during this period from the very late thirties to the late fifties that symptoms of menopausal distress are thought to occur.

The women interviewed in the provincial city had mixed feelings. They felt the obligation to continue "protecting the house" *(katei o mamoru,* which includes all their duties toward the physical house, the social household, and household members) as they were brought up to do, yet they felt dissatisfied with their unproductive days in the house-hold. Many of the informants used menopausal problems as a means of mediating these conflicting feelings, as we shall see below.

In the provincial city, the household is no longer economically impor-tant in a subsistence sense. Economically, it exists for the feeding, sheltering, and nurturance of family members, including sometimes elders. Accordingly, the woman's work in the household is no longer vital for subsistence but only in service to the family's personal needs. It is considered appropriate for subsistence support to come from the man's salary earned outside of the home. (This, of course, does not apply to commercial households that run small shops or traditional craft businesses.) When children are small the woman's productive contribution is not doubted, but as children grow and leave, and if grandparents are living separately,[4] the middle-aged woman herself doubts her productive contribution to the household. Thus, the problem confronting these women in a socioeconomic sense is that their presence in the household is to some extent superfluous in middle age. Work outside the home is possible, but difficult, first, because jobs for women over forty are few in number and poor in quality in this provincial city, and second, because taking jobs feels socially risky. As one of my informants said: "I don't want to go out and wash dishes or clean for someone else. Anyway, if anything would go wrong within the home, it would get blamed on me, the wife. It always does."

Informants' roles in their households continue to be important to them as ways of defining themselves as women and as productive human beings. Some informants cling to their roles as women, mothers, and household co-heads. They have hopes that their children will return to the household, or at least live nearby, and that their meaningful activities within the context of the household and household members will increase.

The middle-aged female informants in this town imparted the idea that the aches and pains they feel in their forties and fifties are largely connected with the menopause, unless other specific medical reasons for these are found. According to the questionnaire, shoulder ache is the most prevalent (21 percent) physical symptom, while dizziness and headache (both 11 percent) are second most prevalent. Almost three-quarters of the women (72 percent) think that menopause is an event that affects a woman both physically and emotionally. Over half (61 percent) feel that they do have emotional symptoms. Among these, irritability *(iraira)* is most prevalent (30.5 percent) and a feeling of having no desire to do anything *(yaruki ga nai)* is second (22 percent).[5]

The questionnaire revealed, however, that a high percentage of women (83 percent) feel that "a woman can control her menopausal problems through mental strength." In conversation this is reflected in the frequently heard statement, "A woman's menopausal problems depend on her *ki* strength." Japanese think that all people have *ki,* an energy that is personal and yet shared with the universe. In a person the energy is both physical and emotional, but in the contemporary colloquial sense, *ki* refers more often to emotional energy. If not controlled, *ki* is an impulsive force that follows one's emotions. If controlled, *ki* is a source of emotional power which is thought to have a strengthening effect for the body and mind; it is the basis of the spiritual energy *(seishin)* used in traditional Japanese arts such as the tea ceremony or the martial arts. In short, women are remarking that if a woman has spiritual energy, or strength of *ki,* to support her body, she will be able to control or overcome her menopausal problems (Rosenberger 1984b).

In the provincial city, three-quarters of the women (76 percent) feel that "Women who are working outside the home have an easier time at menopause." Even though this statement makes "common sense" to informants, women who are not working add in a personal vein that they feel it is better for them to stay home and take care of themselves rather than strain themselves by going to work every day. A few women quit work because of menopausal symptoms, but most working women are satisfied that their work activity does help to prevent menopausal symptoms. Those at home believe that going to work would weaken their general physical and emotional strength so that they might not even be able to perform their basic household tasks. Informants who do not work express the general feelings that they believe are connected with the menopause in terms of their household duties. "I don't even have the will to face making the beds or do the laundry or cook the fish. I just want to go out shopping or talk with my friends. I don't even want to do the things I have to do!"

Women whose activities are mainly limited to the household use menopausal problems to account for the feelings of dissatisfaction with their low level of meaningful activities in the household. They feel dissatisfied, but still want to maintain their central roles in the household and image of devotion to it. They blame their dissatisfaction with the lack of productivity within the household on menopausal symptoms. In short, one way of using menopausal symptoms among informants in the provincial city is as a means of maintaining the woman's necessity to stay at home and of underlining the impossibility of getting a job or engaging in activities outside the home. Excerpts from conversations with several informants illustrate this point.

The first informant is a woman who has never worked outside the home. Unable to have children, she and her husband, an hourly wage worker in a local plant, adopted a relative's child after years of trying. She considers herself "lucky" that her husband and mother-in-law did not force a divorce on her.

> Menopause started for me back in my late thirties. My [adopted] daughter was in junior high school then and I didn't have as much responsibility for her anymore. I got to worrying and thoughts would go round and round in my head. I had headaches and I was so irritable. That was the psychological part of my menopause. You know, they say people who stay in the house too much get menopausal problems. My friends told me I should get out of the house, but I am too weak to hold a job and I have no skills anyway. I started taking tea lessons and being with that group cheered me up. Later, in my forties, I had some of the physical symptoms of menopause.

This woman uses menopausal symptoms as a means of explaining her conflicts with her diminished role in the household and her treatment of menopausal symptoms as a means of explaining her need to get out of the house. As long as these are menopausal problems, her feelings and actions do not represent any rejection of her central role in the household.

I was introduced to this woman by her neighbor, Mrs. Sato, a fifty-year-old woman who had been a key informant over several years. Mrs. Sato, quoted below, was raised in the provincial city but met her husband while teaching school in a country village, where she lived for almost ten years. Her husband is a teacher. At the time of the interviews, Mrs. Sato was teaching one day a week.

> This is the second year of my menopausal problems. They started early for me at forty-seven. I had a bad spell the other day when I was supposed to go with you and my husband out to his home in the country.

(How do you feel when you have a spell?)

> I get into a condition that I just can't express. My shoulders get very stiff, my head hurts, and when I stand, I get dizzy and a bit nauseous. I can't eat, and it does no good to sit or stand. It lasts for a half a day or more and then it just gets better.

(Can you tell when the spells are going to come? Do they have a pattern?)

I'm not quite sure. Sometimes I think that they happen when people are coming to visit. My sister-in-law was supposed to come see me several times recently. The first time I got menopausal problems very badly and had to tell her not to come. When she was to come again, I thought that if I told myself that it was psychological I could overcome my symptoms. But the same thing happened. The symptoms were so bad that I had to cancel the visit. It happened again when two friends were coming to visit and when I was planning to go to a class reunion. Menopausal problems use one's feelings. I feel that I can handle the physical symptoms, but the emotional part—that's frightening, because you're not in control.

My family urges me to go to the doctor, but I tell them that I can figure it out for myself. I understand that the symptoms are menopausal and nobody can cure them anyway. They're natural and will run their course. I just lie here at the *kotatsu* (low warming table). At least I can push the button on the rice cooker for my family's dinner.

During another visit Mrs. Sato said:

I had another really bad spell three weeks ago. I asked the doctor if he didn't think it was menopause, and he said "Well, we'll leave it at that." I think it must be menopause.

Some people tell me that I worry too much about my sons and that's why I get all these menopausal symptoms. My older son has taken a job in Tokyo, but, of course, we hope that he will marry a local girl and come back. I have to be looking for a girl for him to marry soon—before he finds one down there who wouldn't want to live up here. My other son is still in university. I do flower arranging, and we had a trip planned for a night at a hot springs. I think I won't go because my son is taking his exams then. I can't do much for him, but I can at least be here when he comes home.

Sometimes I wish that I had some special accomplishment in life. Maybe that's why I have these menopausal symptoms. My friend who is a professor doesn't have any. On the TV the other day, there was a report on the accomplishments of some students who got the same scholarship that I got when in junior college. I wished that I had accomplished something like that. Now I have these menopausal problems, and I suppose I never will accomplish anything. I'll get better, but never quite the same.

A year later:

> I thought I was an old woman *(obaasan),* but my period came again
> the other week. Just when I was down in Tokyo visiting my eldest son,
> I had one of my attacks in a hotel. I wonder when this will end.

Mrs. Sato's symptoms may be real enough, and they may indeed be
associated with the hormonal changes at menopause, but these questions
are not the subject of this study. Of interest here is that Mrs. Sato uses
her menopausal symptoms as a rationale for staying close to home and
not accomplishing anything more of an individual nature. She takes the
responsibilities of her household (such as being there for her son's exams
and getting a wife for her elder son) quite seriously. As long as she is able
to fulfill those responsibilities, the most basic of which is pressing the
button on the rice cooker, she feels that she is maintaining her position as
a productive member in the household and, in turn, is helping to maintain the household as an active entity. Although her husband says she is
"no longer a woman" since the onset of menopause, she is intent on
keeping her position as mother and household co-head as a means of
maintaining her womanhood as defined by her domestic and productive
labor within the household. Although she says that her husband does
not plan to live with their elder son, she hopes that the elder son and his
future family will be quite near. Mrs. Sato feels some guilt that she is not
"accomplishing" things, but maintenance of her role in the household is
most important. In sum, menopausal symptoms mediate between Mrs.
Sato's desire to maintain her importance as wife and mother in the
household and her realization that she is not using her time for individual accomplishments as some women are.

Another provincial city informant who has never worked outside the
home feels that she has had menopausal symptoms off and on for ten
years.

> I never know when these menopausal symptoms will strike, so I can't
> really plan anything. I have a license for teaching flower arranging,
> but I never know if I will be well enough to teach. I never can plan to
> do anything with my friends either.

> I take hormone shots from the doctor when it gets really bad, because I
> feel that they help me to keep up my body strength so that other
> things don't go wrong. I have to be able at least to cook for my hus-
> band and son, who is in university.

This woman's condition slowly improved over several years. In the last conversation with her, she was quite elated for two reasons: her son had gotten a job locally rather than in Tokyo and her new house with "a kitchen big enough for me and my daughter-in-law" was ready to move into. She has decided she no longer needs hormone shots and is intent on solving any remaining problems through the use of East Asian medicine, which she considers to be less effective but more gentle.

For this informant, menopausal problems have filled the years when her family has dispersed (she has two older daughters as well) and her responsibilities have been few. They allow her to maintain her close relationship with her household not only through her fulfillment of minimal duties, but through her need of household members' sympathy. Although she cannot be assured that, in contemporary Japan, her future daughter-in-law will want to live with her, it is through the possibility of having her household members under one roof that she forsees an end to her menopausal symptoms.

In the provincial city, then, there is a use of menopausal symptoms to mediate or rationalize the conflict that many women feel between the importance of maintaining their position in the household and their lack of productivity in that position. This is not to say that all women in the provincial city suffer inordinately from menopausal symptoms, but vague middle-aged symptoms are attributed to menopause. It is through the association of menopausal symptoms, womanhood, and the woman's role in the household that menopausal symptoms can be said to shore up the household and the middle-aged woman's role in it, both of which have declined in economic importance. In addition, women use menopausal symptoms as a way of mediating, though not really solving, their conflict in giving up individual accomplishments to maintain their central household role. Indeed, for themselves, their womanhood is less threatened by remaining part of the household and by emphasizing the menopausal (thus, female) nature of their middle-aged symptoms.

A few female informants in the provincial city do not use their menopausal symptoms in this way or, in fact, acknowledge menopausal symptoms. One informant, for example, who had come to the provincial city from Tokyo about ten years before, feels that she has overcome her menopausal aches by throwing herself into various hobbies. Another highly educated informant feels that she has overcome the palpitations and nervousness she attributes to the menopause by getting back into her personal research and finally into a job. Another woman, because she is divorced from an alcoholic husband and her job in insurance sales depends on a high level of productivity, has overcome her menopausal symptoms through hormone shots, which she feels to be quick and effective. It is apparent that the three informants discussed here have special attributes: one is an immigrant from Tokyo, another is highly educated, and another is divorced. These informants fit more closely with the ideas and actions about menopause described in the next section.

Refusing the Menopausal Label

In Tokyo, women are in households that, like those in the provincial city, are not economically important for subsistence but function only to service family and personal needs. In contrast to the provincial informants, among the majority of the Tokyo informants, the household as an ideological unit, in which ritual toward ancestors is practiced and in which the co-residence or proximity of parents and elder son's family is stressed, is not of vital importance. Care of the grandparental generation is still a concern, but is done on a more individual, emotional basis: The daughter may care for her own parents, although she is officially in her husband's household, or the son's mother may be taken in when in special need of care. People consider themselves as members of a nuclear family first; their official membership of a household is of less importance.

The middle-aged women interviewed in Tokyo have for the most part completed high school and are married to men who work as salaried workers or professionals. Their orientation could be characterized as more individualistic in relation to their households than the provincial women interviewed. The Tokyo women phrase their problems in middle age not in terms of the decline of the household, but in terms of the difficulty of extracting themselves from family responsibilities or of getting satisfying jobs or activities. Their continuing productive role in the household is not as important to them as is their "role in society." In middle age these women are attracted by a "life of their own," apart from husbands and children. They want to work, have hobbies outside the home, and talk or engage in activities with friends. As a Tokyo woman in her mid-forties said: "Women can't be one-body-one-mind with their husbands anymore. They have to find their 'own world' *(jibun no sekai)*. That's the only way to avoid sinking into the problems of middle age."

Tokyo offers a wider variety of hobbies and jobs than is available in the northeastern provincial city discussed above. There are many community centers where women can learn hobbies such as traditional folk dancing, flower arranging, and ink painting, or more "modern" arts such as jazz dance, oil painting, and paper flower making. In the ink-painting class in which I participated, some women were serious about learning the art, entering their paintings in competitions and even becoming teachers. Other women were there to have a good time with their friends. In both cases, these women in their forties and fifties were attempting to get out of the household and identify themselves as women participating in a nondomestic societal group. Although some were more productive than others, all were participating members of a productive group, something that is evaluated highly in Japanese society. From their own points of view, the women were happy with their involvement in hobbies, giving reasons such as "I can get out of the house and meet with friends," "This gives me enjoyment in my life," and "I am accomplishing something as an individual." They stressed individual enjoyment and accomplishment rather than the productivity of the group. Accordingly, their household roles were maintained to the extent necessary, but not overemphasized.

Japanese women of middle-income families (such as those I interviewed) are increasingly taking employment,[6] and their jobs are becoming part of the basis for their identity. Middle-aged women who have jobs often speak of them as their *ikigai* (meaning in life), especially if those jobs are not absolutely essential for survival but are for their personal satisfaction, to fulfill their need to feel productive and be part of a group outside of the household. Women of middle-income families, in particular, and slightly over half of all women workers are part-time workers.[7] Such hourly, temporary employment is not highly profitable, and part of the money earned usually helps to pay for children's education fees or house loans.[8] However, part of the money earned is pocket money for the woman to buy makeup and clothes or to enjoy a coffee with friends. As one Tokyo woman of forty-five said with a pleased giggle: "My neighbors say they hardly recognize me now as I go off down the street to work—with nice clothes on and my face made up. They say I look ten years younger!"

For the Tokyo informants, jobs and hobbies give alternatives to the productivity—and sexuality—defined by their household roles. Although their productivity is not high as a group of workers and acts to support the mainly male, full-time work force, working informants say that they feel they are contributing to society. More than productivity, women emphasize the rewards for themselves as individuals. These rewards are not measured as much in monetary terms as in terms of a feeling of enjoyment and independence or self-confidence. Informants also feel that their jobs, and to some extent their hobbies, give them the opportunity to make themselves appealing as women again. They remain faithful to their husbands and their household chores, but being out in society allows them to feel the eyes of others evaluating them as women who are still appealing to look at and who are "useful to society." In short, they feel they are beating the image of the dull, middle-aged housewife sitting at home suffering from menopausal symptoms.

The Tokyo informants do not feel that their continued role in the household is necessary to maintain their worth as women, nor do they invest highly in the continuation of the household as an ideological entity. As in the provincial city, the menopausal label is associated with those women whose lives center mainly on the household; three-quarters of the respondents agreed that "menopausal problems will be light for those who work outside of the home."[9] Thus, Tokyo women avoid the menopausal label in order to separate themselves from their household roles and the image of the weakening, aging woman with little productivity or sexuality. They attain a sense of productivity by being part of an extradomestic, productive group and by feeling individual self-confidence. They enhance their sexuality in their own eyes through wearing makeup and fashionable clothes, engaging in independent actions outside the household such as going to coffee houses or night spots with friends, and enjoying repartee with men—actions that provincial city women would avoid. Fashionable urban magazines urge women to enjoy their sexuality with husbands or lovers: "The menopausal years are the peak of the woman's sex urge" (Okifuji 1982). Tokyo women argue that the presence or absence of menstruation and reproductive capability has nothing to do with sexual attractiveness (despite instances of husbands who mourn the end of menstruation as the fading of the sexual appeal of their wives). By partially detaching themselves from their responsibilities in the household, by engaging in activities "in society," and by avoiding the menopausal label, these *modaan* (modern) middle-aged women emphasize both their usefulness as people and their womanhood, independent of their household roles.

When Tokyo informants have physical or psychological complaints, they try to deemphasize menopause as the cause of their problems because of the image of nonproductivity and loss of sexuality that the label "menopausal problems" *(kōnenki shōgai)* carries (Rosenberger 1984a, chap. 11). Only one-third of Tokyo informants agreed with a statement that "It is natural that in the menopausal years women suffer physical symptoms." They preferred to label their physical problems as "aging phenomena." However, three-quarters agreed that "It is natural that in the menopausal period women suffer irritability and psychological instability." Thus, these women emphasize the emotional nature of their problems during middle age. They hesitate to call them "menopausal problems," and prefer instead to label them as "neuroses" or "syndromes."

Mrs. Tsuda, a fifty-year-old woman I interviewed at a Tokyo checkup clinic, was in the midst of the dilemma of how to extract herself from her responsibilities to her family and get back to her job. She is a professional woman who has already rejected "menopausal" as a label for her difficulties. But her words show her indecision about how to account for and solve her problems outside of that label.

> I've never really had menopausal problems. My period has been finished for about one year now. I didn't worry much about it when it was irregular; I thought it was to be expected so I didn't go to the doctor. After that, I had some psychological problems, not because of menopause, but because of my age. My ability to be patient went down and I've gotten selfish. I got sick of housework; I call it a "housewife syndrome."

> *(What do you think caused your psychological problems?)*

> Ever since university I've been in radio announcing. I quit for awhile because I kept having miscarriages and the doctor said there was too much stress. You have to work odd hours. But now that the children are older—they're sixteen and twenty-five—I want to be freer to do my work as I please. But my son, the 25-year-old, still lives with us even though he has a job. When he got a job, I strongly suggested to him that he move out, but he's still there. It's convenient for him because he likes to spend his money on concerts. Of course, I still have to do his laundry and make his meals. I get so irritated.

This Tokyo woman prefers to label her "psychological problems" as "housewife syndrome" rather than as "menopausal problems." She brushes off talk of menopause with a short account of menses irregularity and cessation "just as was to be expected." At the beginning of the interview Mrs. Tsuda did not want to blame her problems on her family members. Her first reaction was to blame the problem on her own psychological inadequacies and label them as a syndrome or neurosis. Later in the conversation, Mrs. Tsuda admitted to what she thinks is the one real cause of her "psychological problems": her son's not moving out even though he has a job. Her husband does not urge the son to move out. She thinks that her household responsibilities are taking time from her career just when she should be getting free of her housewifely chores.

Mrs. Tsuda is unwilling to disguise her problems as menopausal problems, but she is hesitant to do anything about the causes of her dissatisfaction, although she has formed a group of working women friends that get together to talk about their problems. She has not yet gone to a psychiatrist or counselor for help, but feels relieved to talk to a doctor (an internist at the hospital where we met), who agrees that her problem is a type of neurosis.

Japanese women like Mrs. Tsuda are differentiating their domestic problems from their "menopausal problems." By explaining their problems as neuroses or syndromes, they accept a large degree of personal responsibility and try to solve their problems through their own actions without demanding change from family members.

A popular book published in 1982 outlines the woman's adult life in terms of a series of syndromes. The author, a woman, writes, "It's easy to overlook the 'empty-nest syndrome' or the 'husband-hating syndrome' because such syndromes occur at the same time of life as menopausal problems" (Fukuda 1982, 142). She urges her readers to take action that will change their domestic situations. "Rebel against your husband. Don't help. Play hookey from your housework. Sleep late on Sundays" (Fukuda 1982, 143). The content of her advice addresses one of the main problems of those middle-aged Japanese women with an orientation toward their own individual accomplishments. And yet by her consistent use of the suffix for syndrome *(shō)*, the author poses women's problems as though they are medical problems.

The Tokyo woman of fifty quoted below described her unique set of problems. In interview, she refused to write her problems off as menopausal symptoms, but at the same time she voiced her confusion as to how to handle them: Should she deal with them as part of a neurosis or use them as motivation for divorce?

I've just turned fifty. These turning points are so difficult. At forty I was tired of taking care of a small child while I worked. But now things are worse. My period is irregular and I've got more worries.

(What kind of worries?)

My joints ache and my period keeps stopping. That's menopausal problems, I know. I did Chinese exercises and got my period going again. But then it stopped again because of a shocking event in my life. After that I couldn't sleep for forty days. I wanted to get out and wander around, it was so bad. I really felt like I wanted to die. I don't think that's menopausal distress. I think it has to do with my psychological worries. It's a kind of neurosis.

(Do you still work?)

No. I continued until about three years ago, but it was too hard to commute. You see, about six years ago, my husband built a house a couple of hours out of Tokyo. He built it with our money without even asking me. He insisted we all move out there, even though I prefer the city where I was raised.

(Can't you go back to work?)

Well, to tell you the truth, when my son was in ninth grade—three years ago—he got into some trouble. I had always been the kind to let him do as he likes, so his father blamed it on me. He wants me to stay home now for our son. But our son is already separated from us even though he lives with us. If only I could work, it would be all right. But my husband gives me no understanding. I wonder if I'm going crazy when I can't sleep and forget to turn off the gas. Then I feel anxious about my health because I'm not having my period.

(And then you have to worry whether you're pregnant or not, I suppose.)

On, no, there's no worry about that. We've had no sexual relations for six years, ever since I found out about the house. I can't trust him anymore.

Mrs. Sakai illustrates the confusion of an educated, work-oriented, middle-aged woman in the early 1980s. Her resistance to labeling all her symptoms as "menopausal problems" is directly related to her sharp disagreement with her husband's ideas that the household should be her central concern and that she should be responsible for her son (who will carry on the household).

She realizes that some of her symptoms are the result of her dissatisfaction with her life. Although she calls her psychological symptoms a neurosis, she really believes that her mental state is caused by her husband's actions and attitude. She tries to distract herself by meeting with her friends, hiking in the mountains, and doing calligraphy, but she wants to work and thus have the possibility of economic independence, however unstable. Unable to separate from her husband, she refuses to have a sexual relationship as a sign of her dissatisfaction.

An increasing number of women in the menopausal years are getting divorced.[10] The reason is not only that husbands think women in the menopausal years are aging and losing their sexual attractiveness. Women want to "try their wings" *(tonde iru onna)* without husbands looking on. A sign of women's increasing bid for change in the household is men's increasing discomfort with the household. Newspapers, books, and magazines are focusing on men's uncertainty with their lives. Japanese women themselves sometimes comment that men are even more pitiful than women.[11] As one woman put it: "We have it bad. But men have it worse. We at least have time to think about having a fulfilled life. Men just have to go to work everyday and do what they're told. They're not allowed to stop because then the money stops. They're the ones that are getting 'menopausal problems' now, not the women!"

Conclusion

The decline of the economic and ideological importance of the Japanese household interweaves with the ways menopausal problems are used by middle-aged Japanese women. The reason for this intertwining is that the place of Japanese women in the household as wife, mother, subsistence laborer, and domestic nurturer has been and to some extent is an important part of the definition of the female gender. Middle-aged women use ideas and actions about menopausal problems to control their image in relation to the household.

In the farming-fishing community, where the household is still economically important, women use menopausal problems to emphasize their devotion as mother and worker to the household regardless of whether they are disowning or claiming menopausal problems for themselves. In the provincial city, where the household is still ideologically but no longer economically important, many women use menopausal problems as a way of mediating their conflict between wanting to maintain the integrity of the household and their roles in it and wanting to find some individual expression outside of it. In Tokyo many educated women use a denial of menopause to emphasize their independence from the household. They see themselves as "people in society" and promote their definition of women through their sexual attractiveness, self-fulfillment, and independence.

The progression of this chapter shows that Japanese women are breaking away from the traditional ideology of the household and women's identity with the household in middle age. This is not to say that women's reproductive and domestic labor has become irrelevant in Japan; indeed, within the context of the gender relations upon which economic production depends in Japan, women's labor within the home is essential, especially because of the long hours worked by Japanese salaried men and the emphasis on achievement through tests for children. The "free time" *(hima)* that middle-aged women experience between their late thirties (when their children are in school) and their mid-fifties (when their husbands retire) is only relative and comes at a time when women are discriminated against for jobs of higher skill and higher pay.[12] The break from traditional household ideology is not manifested in an increase of women's status and productivity in the extradomestic world, although it is manifested in an increase in the number of women working.

What is significant in women's shift away from identity with the household and toward a stronger identity with society outside the household is that women of middle age are striving to express and enjoy their individuality. The middle-class women interviewed in Tokyo are not so concerned with proving their maturity through complete devotion to an extradomestic productive group as they are with indulging their individual tastes. Women fulfill the minimum necessary tasks at home and they usually follow the appropriate channels of work or hobbies outside the household, but extradomestic tasks are done with a relish, for enjoyment, and often for the purpose of having a sense of individual "worth in life."

I would suggest that middle-aged women who are breaking away from the traditional ideology of the household constitute a group that is in the forefront of a new definition of the individual in Japan. They are flirting with individualism and democracy as it was defined by the Japanese after World War II: "do-as-you-like-ism." Young people also fit this description, but the case of middle-aged women is more startling because they are supposed to be "mature" and in control of their individual spirits that lead them to indulgence. Although middle-aged women are not openly advocating their own ideas about more personal freedom, their actions and attitudes are a subtle challenge to the notion of adult maturity as controlled self-discipline. They are asking if the definition of maturity must be confined to the devotion of self to the tasks of the group, if the definition of maturity can include the expression of individual will with friends and in the informal practice of individual interests.

Middle-aged women are the main group of mature adults in Japan that have the free time to "indulge" themselves in such questions. Although middle-aged males often make fun of their wives as "always playing" (at hobbies or jobs), these wives are slowly giving new legitimacy to the idea that work and hobbies can be enjoyed because they are pleasurable and because they give personal meaning. A woman in her late thirties looking for a job said, "Women can't be like men, who will do any job for the money. For we women, a little money is important for a feeling of independence, but if we don't find meaning in the job, we don't do it." These middle-aged women are not the nonconformists or emotional purists (Lebra 1976, 161) revered by Japanese for their self-restraint. They are mature adults, in control of their *ki,* and who are unabashedly interested in investing themselves in friendships and activities that center around their enjoyment as individuals.

This ideology of enjoyment and accomplishment for self causes consternation among provincial city women. It is they who are defending and rationalizing their need to devote themselves to their traditional household roles while Tokyo women are feeling little or no need to defend their extradomestic actions. A provincial city woman in her mid-thirties showed the increasing difficulty of her traditional role as a daughter-in-law in her husband's household.

My parents-in-law expect me to do everything for them without as much as a thank-you. I even had to say I was coming to confer about my daughter's English lessons to come here and talk this afternoon. I get so jealous of my friends who are now getting free of household duties and starting to take jobs or do hobbies. Sometimes I think I should get divorced.

This woman's thoughts of divorce were quickly squelched by her older neighbor, at whose house we were talking, but the younger woman's words are an indication of the changing attitude among the next generation of middle-aged provincial city women. They will not cling to the household and its responsibilities as the nexus of their womanhood and activity, as their elders have. Thus, the variation among middle-aged women found in Japan of the early 1980s reflected in this study will decrease in the future as more women refuse the menopausal label associated with a traditional household orientation.

Women such as Mrs. Sakai, the Tokyo woman quoted in the previous section, are beginning to view, and be encouraged to understand, their problems of interrelationships within the household in a more straightforward manner, rather than disguising them as medical problems such as menopausal symptoms or neuroses. Middle-aged women in the larger cities are increasingly unwilling to constrain their lives to the social structure of the household because it has little meaning for them as an ideological entity. Lebra (1984, 295) argues that Japanese women live their lives according to the constraints of the social structure, and indeed middle-aged women in the fishing-farming village and the provincial city still live according to the constraints of the household and sometimes try to preserve these constraints even when they are falling away. However, the tendency in the larger cities is toward an increasing unwillingness for women past the childbearing years (over thirty-five) to constrain themselves to the needs of the household and its members. Even in the provincial city the idea of achieving individual fulfillment and enjoyment in the midst of mature female adulthood is rarely any longer labeled "selfish" *(wagamama)*. As a provincial woman in her early forties said, "Children are not a life theme. I want to find a theme for myself, for my own life."

Japanese adult men, too, will be influenced by the changing ideas about adult maturity. Even now, men are said to have "menopausal problems" if they suffer from physical or psychological symptoms that are thought to stem from too much stress from the work situation. They are urged by doctors, wives, and journalists to relax with their friends and their hobbies *(Jidai* 1981). Individual enjoyment is being urged upon mature middle-aged men at the "peak of their working life" *(hatarakizakari)*. The conflict between status and individual enjoyment is greater for middle-aged Japanese men than Japanese women, although the conflict may decrease as postwar babies reach middle age.[13]

In part these ideas of a decrease in middle-aged status and an increase in individual enjoyment for men as well as the increased employment for middle-aged women (defined as individual enjoyment) are necessary ideological corollaries to the needs of the Japanese economy. Large companies are overflowing with high-status middle managers (Nihon Keizai Shimbunsha 1984) and promotion is difficult; the majority of middle-aged men will not find high status through their jobs, and individual enjoyment is an alternative to the failing Japanese promise. A large group of part-time laborers who can be laid off is now necessary to the Japanese economy, and middle-aged women, who find flexibility in hours and ease in quitting to their liking, are a favored group of workers for opportunistic hiring and firing.

Conflict will come, both at home and at work, if large numbers of women begin to demand full-time, secure employment with promotions. My prediction is that this will not happen soon because of the continuing high value put on male status, motherhood, and the education of the children. Women of middle age and most younger women are not seriously challenging the differences in gender status between men and women; they are only claiming their rights to use their free time as independent individuals.

Notes

1. Records show that in the 1800s and early 1900s, the girl's first menstruation was celebrated by distributing red rice to neighbors and friends, as well as by eating red rice at a family party. The red of the rice corresponded to the sun. Such celebrations were reported by middle-aged informants raised in the country. In the early 1980s a television advertisement for tampons in Japan showed a high school student buying her tampons and then bowing to the sun on the old-style Japanese flag.

2. In 1981 the average age at marriage for men and women was 25.3 years of age. The majority of women are now marrying between 20 and 24 years of age. Because the average age for having a first child is between 24 and 25 now and was between 22 and 23 for the middle-aged generation, mothers are usually in their late forties before their daughters bear children. The majority of men marry between 25 and 29, so that the children of the first male son (the "inner" grandchildren, who by law belong to the same household as the grandparents) are usually not born until the grandmother is into her fifties.

The birth rate has decreased from 36 births per 1,000 population in 1920, to 26 in 1939, to 17–18 in 1955; it steadied at 18 births per 1,000 population in the

1970s (Suzuki and Ishikawa 1974, 9). In 1978 the birth rate was 14.9 births per 1,000 people and in 1982 it was the lowest in history, 12.9 per 1,000 (*Asahi Shimbun*, Jan. 1, 1983).

3. Average age of menstrual cessation (Hirano, Tsukada, Honda 1979, 14):

Year	Age
1964	48.4
1971	49.8
1979	52.0

4. The percentage of people over sixty-five living in three-generation households has decreased from 54.4 percent in 1975 to 50.1 percent in 1980, to 48.9 percent in 1982 (*Asahi Shimbun*, Jan. 3, 1983). Some women who do not live with their sons or daughters but live nearby care for the grandchildren if the daughter or daughter-in-law has a job.

5. In the questionnaire survey conducted in the provincial city, respondents were asked to list any physical and emotional symptoms that they associated with the menopause. A list of symptoms was not given. All respondents were between the ages of thirty and sixty. Three-quarters of the 189 respondents were attenders of a community-sponsored exercise class. The remaining quarter were women whom the researcher met through an introduction from doctors and from key female informants.

6. Middle-income families are defined by their husband's income: between 3.88 million yen ($15,520) and 5.01 million yen ($20,040). From 1981 to 1983 employment of wives of middle income families rose from 37.9 percent to 45.1 percent. The rise was "attributed . . . to an increase in the number of women working part time" (*Japan Times*, Oct. 16, 1983).

7. Slightly over half of all women workers are part-time workers. Part-time workers sometimes work forty hours a week, but they are not official members of the company and are paid hourly wages. They may be laid off at the will of the company; lay-offs were increasing in the early 1980s with the increased use of robot automation (*Asahi Shimbun*, Feb. 13, 1983), as well as the sluggish economy. About one-third of women workers work at family businesses or farms.

8. About half of women workers say that they work to "make money to keep the household going (especially for housing loans and children's education)." The second and third most frequent reasons for working are "because it's the household's business" and "because I have free time." About 20 percent of women say they work for reasons such as "work is my meaning in life *(ikigai)*" or "I want to develop my self" (*Nihon Rōmu Kenkyūkai* 1984, 183–184).

9. The Tokyo questionnaire survey asked for a positive to negative response (1–4) on various ideas about menopause and menopausal symptoms. Although some questions were the same as in the provincial city questionnaire, the format was different. Respondents were one hundred women who were interviewed as they came into a yearly checkup clinic in a mid-sized Tokyo hospital.

10. There is a new peak in divorce statistics for people in their late forties and early fifties. Many of these divorces are being initiated by women. According to the Ministry of Health and Welfare, 22.2 percent of the wives who got divorced in 1981 were over forty, and 30.9 percent of the husbands who got divorced in 1981 were over forty. In 1982 the divorce rate in Japan was 1.40 couples per 1,000 population. (It was 5.3 for the U.S. in 1982.) Of the couples divorced, the percentage that had been together for at least ten years before divorce was 35 percent in 1981, and 38.6 percent in 1982 (*Asahi Shimbun,* Jan. 1, 1983). Women who get divorced in Japan rarely get remarried.

11. In a recent survey of men's and women's feelings about the nuclear family, men showed greater dissatisfaction than women. More than wives, husbands felt their feelings did not fit with the rest of the family, that they did not have a place to be when at home, and that they could not rest at home.

12. Many jobs, even for supermarket chain checkout girls (such as in Kinokuniya), are given only to women under thirty-five, and even then good looks is part of the hiring policy. Young women are also discriminated against for promotion and encouraged to quit by their late twenties, although 60 percent of large companies now have the policy that women can be employed and promoted as lifetime employees. Women who are teachers can reenter the system only as part-time teachers (who are rare) once they have quit. Nurses can get jobs after raising children, but only at the smaller, less well paying hospitals.

13. A book put out by the Japan Economic Newspaper called *Nihon no midoru (Japan's middle management)* reports that middle managers in their thirties prefer to spend their after-hours with colleagues of the same age. They are less bent on achieving status, especially through involvement with the vertical hierarchy of the company at a time when they feel they deserve their individual enjoyment.

References

Bachnik, J. 1983. Recruitment and strategies for household succession. *Man* 18:160–182.

Bart, Pauline. 1969. Why women's status changes in middle age. *Sociological Symposium* 3:1–18.

Beyene, Y. 1984. Cultural significance and physiological manifestation of menopause. MS.

Brown, J. 1982. Cross-cultural perspectives on middle-aged women. *Current Anthropology* 23:143–148.

Brown, K. 1966. *Dōzoku* and the ideology of descent in rural Japan. *American Anthropologist* 68:1129–1151.

Caudill, W. 1962. Patterns of emotion in modern Japan. In *Japanese culture,* ed. R. J. Smith and R. K. Beardsley. Chicago: Aldine.

Davis, D. L. 1982. *Blood and nerves.* Social and Economic Studies No. 28.

188   *Nancy R. Rosenberger*

Memorial University of Newfoundland Institute of Social and Economic Research.

Flint, M. 1979. Transcultural influences in peri-menopause. In *Psychosomatics in peri-menopause*, ed. I. Haspels, A. H. Musaph, and H. Heymann. Baltimore: University Park Press.

Fukuda, K. 1982. Ryōsai Kenbo o osou "Shufushōkōgun" no fukimi na ryūkō (The strange popularity of the "Housewife Syndrome" which attacks the Good Wife and Wise Mother). *Shūkan Asahi* 310:141–143.

Hirano, M., I. Tsukada, and H. Honda. 1979. *Sanfujinka shikkan no kiso chishiki* (Basic knowledge of gynecological complaints). Tokyo: Medical Research Center.

Jidai. 1981. Natsu ni zokuhatsu suru otoko no "kōnenki shōgai" okuriya suru (Getting rid of men's menopausal problems that originate in summer). 9:87–91.

Kawashima, K. 1978. *Josei no karada—haha to musume no tame ni* (Women's bodies—for mothers and daughters). Tokyo: Shinko Koeki Isho Shuppankyoku.

Kitaoji, H. 1971. Structure of the Japanese family. *American Anthropologist* 73:1036–1057.

Lebra, T. 1976. *Japanese patterns of behavior.* Honolulu: Univ. of Hawaii Press.

———. 1984. *Japanese women.* Honolulu: Univ. of Hawaii Press.

Lock, M. 1986 Ambiguities of aging. *Culture, Medicine and Psychiatry* 10:23–46.

Madoka, Y. 1982. *Shufushōkōgun* (The housewife syndrome). Tokyo: Bunda Shuppankyoku.

Moaz, B., et al. 1970. Female attitudes to menopause. *Social Psychiatry* 1:35–40.

Nakane, C. 1970. *Japanese society.* Berkeley and Los Angeles: Univ. of California Press.

Nihon Keizai Shimbunsha. 1984. *Nihon no midoru* (Japan's middle management). Tokyo.

Nihon Rōmu Kenkyūkai. 1984. *Rōmu nenkan* (Labor yearbook). Tokyo.

Ohnuki-Tierney, E. 1984. *Illness and culture in contemporary Japan.* Cambridge: Cambridge Univ. Press.

Okifuji, N. 1982. *Onna wa rōgo hitori de kurasō* (Women, let's live our old age alone). *Fujin Koron* 1:192–199.

Rosenberger, N. R. 1984a. Middle-aged Japanese women and the meaning of the menopausal transition. Ph.D. diss. University of Michigan.

———. 1984b. The uncontrolled *ki*. Paper presented at the annual Association for Asian Studies meeting, Mar. 23–25, Washington, D.C.

Suzuki, M., and H. Ishikawa. 1974. *Kōnenki shōgai* (Climacteric disturbance). Tokyo: Igaku Shoin.

Smith, R. J. 1983. *Japanese Society.* Cambridge: Cambridge Univ. Press.

CONTRIBUTORS

Christie W. Kiefer is associate professor of anthropology at the University of California, San Francisco, where he teaches in both the Development and Aging and the Medical Anthropology programs. He has written on Japanese personality and social change, on aging among Japanese and Korean Americans, and on the cultural aspects of aging in general.

Margaret Lock received her Ph.D. in cultural anthropology from the University of California, Berkeley. She is currently professor of medical anthropology in the Department of Humanities and Social Studies in Medicine and the Department of Anthropology, McGill University. She is past-president of the Society for Medical Anthropology and author of *East Asian Medicine in Urban Japan: Varieties of Medical Experience* and numerous articles on medical anthropology with an emphasis on Japan.

Susan Orpett Long, who holds a doctorate from the University of Illinois, teaches anthropology and East Asian studies at John Carroll University. She has published numerous articles on the Japanese medical system and its cultural context and is author of *Family Change and the Life Course in Japan.*

Edward Norbeck, who was educated at the University of Michigan, is currently professor of anthropology (emeritus) at Rice University. He is the author or editor of thirteen books and many articles. Among his publications are *Changing Japan* and *From Country to City: Takashima Urbanized.*

David K. Reynolds was formerly on the faculties of the University of California, Los Angeles, the University of Southern California Medical School, and the University of Houston. At present he is director of the

ToDo Institute in Los Angeles and codirector of the Health Center Pacific, Maui. He has written fifteen books on Japan, the Japanese, and mental health topics, among them, *The Quiet Therapies: Japanese Pathways to Personal Growth.*

Nancy R. Rosenberger is presently a Mellon Postdoctoral Fellow in Asian Studies at Emory University, where she is affiliated with the Department of Anthropology. She received her Ph.D. from the University of Michigan with a dissertation on middle-aged women and the ideology of menopause in Japan. She is currently working on a book on self, power, and gender in Japan.

William E. Steslicke is associate professor of health policy and management in the College of Public Health, University of South Florida. He holds a Ph.D. in political science from the University of Illinois. In 1982 he was a visiting associate of the Institute of Public Health in Tokyo. He has published numerous articles on health care organization and policies in Japan and is author of *Doctors in Politics: The Political Life of the Japan Medical Association.*

AUTHOR INDEX

SUBJECT INDEX

Minamata disease, 25
Ministry of Education, Science, and Culture, 75, 113; and school health programs, 36
Ministry of Finance, 37
Ministry of Health and Welfare (MHW/ Kōseishō), 54, 56, 75, 113, 187n.10; and care for elderly, 93; and medical care policy controversy, 57, 58, 59; National Health Survey of, 30–34, 38; organization and activities, 36, 37, 50
Ministry of International Trade and Industry (MITI), 55
Ministry of Justice, 113
Ministry of Welfare (prewar), 35
Minkan katsuryoku ("the vitality of the private sector"), 59
Minsei-iin (lay social workers), 97
Mishima Yukio, 135
Modernization: convergence model of, x, 17, 84–85; illness associated with, 16
Morbidity indicators (National Health Survey), 30–34
Morioka city, 95, 96
Morita therapy, 115, 118, 120, 121–122, 123, 125, 126, 127
Mortality, 26–30; infant, 4, 27, 28 (table), 95, 96; leading causes of, 27, 28 (table), 29; suicide, 4, 9, 27, 28, 29 (table), 30 (table), 135, 136
Mother, illnesses caused by *(bogenbyō)*, 144–146
Mother-in-law, 167, 171; position in traditional family, 148, 164
"Moving-day depression," 131, 143–144
Moxibustion, 34, 66, 104, 110, 130
"Muntera" (unskilled chatting), 118
Musashino: geriatric care system in, 94–95
Musculoskeletal system diseases, 31, 32, 34

Nagasaki: Dutch studies at, 70, 71, 73
Naikan therapy, 112, 118, 119–120, 122, 123, 125, 126, 127
Nakai, 112
National Health Insurance Law of 1958, 46, 58
National Health Survey (Kokumin Kenkō Chōsa), 30–34, 38
National Police Agency: data on suicide, 28, 30
Natural food, 132
Neo-Confucian medicine, 68–69
Nephritis, 27

Nervous system diseases, 31, 32, 34
Netakiri ("bedridden"), 103
Neurosis/Neurotic depression, 12, 16, 114, 115–116, 122, 123, 125, 126, 131; menopause as, 178, 179, 180, 181
Nihonjinron, 16
Ningen jōhatsu ("human evaporation"), 134
Nishizono, (M.), 112
Nonconformism, 134, 183
Nonspecific complaints, 13, 138, 140–142, 143, 145
Nursery schools, 145
Nurses, 187n.12; education and licensure of, 40, 41; number and distribution, 42, 78; percentage of women as, 79–80
Nursing homes, 11, 92, 93, 101, 107; associated with poverty, 102; number of beds and homes, 90, 94
Nurturance, 5, 9, 104, 105, 151

"Obaasute-yama" ("Granny-flinging Mountain"), 105
Occupation: health and welfare during, 35–36, 37
Office of the Prime Minister, 37
Ōgata Kōan, 86n.10
Okamoto Kozo, 135
Okonogi, (K.), 112
Old Age Health Act, 93
Ossipov, A. N., ix

Paramedical workers/Technicians, 40–41, 77–81, 83, 102
Parent abuse by children, 16, 125
Passivity. See Dependency
"Path of blood" *(chi no michi):* origin of term, 164
Pfizer Taito Company, 51
Pharmaceutical Affairs Bureau, 50
Pharmaceutical industry, 151; production and sales, 51–54; profits by 16 companies, 53
Pharmacists: education and licensure of, 40, 80; number, 42, 78 (table); women as, 79–80
Physician(s): dominance of medical care system by, 39, 43, 78, 79–82, 83; education and licensure of, 39–40, 42, 43, 68–69, 70, 71, 72, 73, 74, 78, 80, 81–82, 85n.1, 85n.3, 86n.9; government support for, 74–75, 79; and *ikyoku* system, 81–82; membership in JMA, 86n.11; number and dis-